Desire
and Passion

The Ultimate Guide to Boosting Libido and Finding Fulfilled Love

By
Dr. Lucas Berger

Desire and Passion

The Ultimate Guide to Boosting Libido and Finding Fulfilled Love

Table of Contents

Introduction

In the intricate dance of intimacy, desire often plays the role of the elusive partner. It's a force that drives us to seek connection, yet can be as fleeting as a whisper. The journey to rekindling this passion is not just one of the body, but of the mind and spirit as well. This book seeks to guide you through that journey, offering practical tools and expert insights designed to enhance your libido and deepen your connection with your partner.

Desire is an ever-evolving element in our lives, shaped by a myriad of factors including emotional states, physical health, and life circumstances. It is dynamic, capable of waxing and waning, demanding attention, understanding, and sometimes, a little coaxing back to life. This book doesn't promise a quick fix—rather, it opens avenues for exploration and renewal, encouraging a holistic approach to embracing and enhancing desire.

One of the foundational aspects of this exploration is understanding. Why does desire dwindle? What can reignite it? We delve into the science behind libido, debunking common myths and establishing facts that may challenge conventional wisdom. You'll discover that desire isn't simply a biological response, but an intricate interplay of physical, emotional, and relational factors.

Central to the awakening of desire is communication and connection. Nothing thrives in isolation, and desire is no different. We explore the importance of open dialogue, equipping you with techniques for effective communication that foster a nurturing environment for intimacy. You'll learn that words—both spoken and unspoken—carry immense power in shaping desire.

Physical well-being also significantly influences libido. The book sheds light on how exercise can restore balance and stimulate desire, introducing specific types of activities that could energize your libido. Whether it's the uplifting power of cardiovascular training or the strength-building rewards of weight lifting, physical fitness forms a crucial pillar in this multifaceted approach to intimacy.

But the path to a vibrant libido isn't trodden by physical fitness alone. Nutrition plays a vital role, and you will uncover the foods and supplements that are allies in enhancing your desire. Essential vitamins and minerals, along with herbal remedies, are explored for their libido-boosting properties, offering you a natural route to well-being.

Emotional intimacy serves as a bridge to physical desire. In these pages, you will find insights into building trust and vulnerability, crucial components of a thriving intimate relationship. Learning to share feelings openly, practicing empathy, and providing emotional support can create an environment where desire naturally flourishes.

The obstacles to an active libido often lie in everyday life's stressors and challenges. From managing work-life balance to employing stress reduction techniques, we offer strategies for overcoming these common barriers. Understanding how to navigate these hurdles will empower you to reclaim your desire and intimacy.

Touch and sensuality can be transformative, awakening dormant desires and creating profound connections. Learn the art of sensual massage and the importance of exploring and utilizing erogenous zones as part of a fulfilling intimate experience. Rediscover the power of touch in nurturing your relationship and igniting your passion.

This book also addresses practical aspects of sexual techniques and practices, providing guidance on enhancing pleasure. Whether it's trying new positions or understanding the nuances of foreplay, these practices are shared with a focus on mutual enjoyment and the importance of playfulness in desire.

Long-term relationships demand continuous nurturing to keep the spark alive. Discover romantic gestures and surprises that celebrate your union, infused with creativity and love. From planning date nights to spontaneous acts of love, these romantic endeavors can reinforce and rejuvenate your connection.

Mental health cannot be overlooked when exploring libido. Addressing issues such as depression and anxiety is crucial for a healthy desire. The book discusses therapy options and support techniques, encouraging you to seek help when needed and recognizing the profound impact mental well-being has on intimacy.

Lifestyle choices, too, affect intimacy. We examine the impact of smoking, alcohol, and drug use on desire, and share strategies for promoting positive lifestyle changes. This awareness enables you to make informed decisions that can enhance rather than diminish your libido.

Throughout the journey, hormonal imbalances can present unique challenges. Understanding these influences allows for effective treatments, ranging from medical interventions to natural alternatives. By gaining insight into hormonal balance, you can make informed choices about your health and sexual desire.

Additionally, real-life success stories and insights from sex therapists provide inspiration and practical advice. These narratives remind us of the shared human experience, offering lessons and validated techniques that have stood the test of time and investigation.

The role of technology in modern relationships is explored, highlighting both opportunities and challenges for intimacy in the digital age. Managing screen time, balancing technology with relationship needs, and using digital communication tools wisely can enhance rather than hinder your intimate connections.

Desire evolves as we age, influenced by different life stages such as young adulthood, parenthood, and beyond. This book offers strategies for maintaining passion throughout these transitions, ensuring that your libido keeps pace with your changing life.

Cultural and societal influences on libido are also addressed, encouraging media literacy and self-acceptance strategies that bolster a positive body image. This fosters an environment where desire can thrive, free from unrealistic expectations and pressures.

Ultimately, this book is an invitation to explore your own fantasies and desires, safely and openly. Communication of boundaries and establishing comfort zones allows for free exploration, making these personal journeys enriching and exhilarating.

Understanding sexuality and gender differences is crucial for a comprehensive view of desire. Respecting individual differences and adopting inclusive approaches lay the groundwork for mutual understanding and a deeply fulfilling intimate relationship.

Planned adventures and novelty add an exciting dimension to desire. By trying new activities together, spicing up routines with adventurous dates, or embracing novel experiences, you can rediscover the joy and thrill of intimacy.

Even in long-distance relationships, intimacy can thrive. Creative solutions and virtual date ideas help maintain connection and love across miles, allowing your relationship to flourish despite physical separation.

If you've experienced a breakup or crisis, this book guides you toward healing and rekindling passion. With steps for rebuilding trust and navigating grief, these strategies provide hope and a pathway forward.

Celebrating love and milestones reflects continuity and commitment. Planning celebrations and marking important dates affirm your journey together, creating long-lasting memories and reinforcing your bond.

This book serves as your companion in understanding and enhancing desire. Embrace the journey, support each other, and discover the profound depths of connection and intimacy awaiting you.

Chapter 1:
Understanding Desire and Passion

In the symphony of human connection, desire and passion play the crescendo that turns a mere melody into an unforgettable masterpiece. They are the twin forces that fuel our intimate relationships, driving us to seek deeper bonds and a more fulfilling love life. Understanding desire isn't just about decoding the science behind libido or debunking myths—it's about acknowledging the tapestry of emotions, fantasies, and connections that make us feel alive. Passion, on the other hand, is the spark that kindles our hearts and whispers possibilities, urging us to explore the depths of our yearnings with fervent curiosity. It's an intimate dance between partners, where vulnerability meets strength, and connection transcends the ordinary. This journey invites us to embrace our authentic selves and engage with our partners on a richer, more profound level, setting the stage for the chapters that follow in this exploration of love and intimacy.

The Science Behind Libido

Libido, often defined as sexual desire or drive, is a complex interplay of human physiology, psychology, and myriad external influences. To understand libido deeply, it's essential to delve into its multifaceted nature, the roles played by various hormones, and the impact of both the mind and body. This section aims to illuminate the science behind libido, enabling you to appreciate the underlying factors contributing to this vital aspect of intimate relationships.

At its core, libido is fueled by hormonal activity. Testosterone, primarily known as a male hormone, is crucial for libido in all genders. It influences not only physical arousal but also the capacity to foster desire and sustain it over time. Meanwhile, estrogen and progesterone contribute significantly in differing ways, affecting libido cycles, particularly in women. During times of hormonal fluctuation, such as menstruation or menopause, libido can markedly change, highlighting the dynamic nature of this drive.

Yet, hormones don't work in isolation. Dopamine, a neurotransmitter, plays a vital role in the brain's reward system and is intimately linked with arousal. When one experiences pleasure, dopamine levels rise, reinforcing behaviors that lead to this state. Similarly, oxytocin, known as the "love hormone," fosters intimacy, bonding, and heightened sexual desire. It's often released in abundance during physical touch or orgasm, reinforcing emotional closeness and attraction between partners.

The psychological dimension of libido is equally significant. Stress, anxiety, and depression can dampen sexual desire through complex biochemical pathways that affect neurotransmitter activity. Cortisol, the stress hormone, can inhibit the production and action of sexual hormones, thereby diminishing libido. On the other hand, relaxation and mental well-being can promote an increase in sexual desire by creating an environment where the mind is open to pleasure and connection.

The brain, often described as the largest sex organ, is instrumental in mediating libido through mental imagery and erotic fantasies. It initiates arousal and modulates desire through the interplay of thoughts, emotions, and perceptions. Positive body image and feelings of self-worth are crucial psychological components that can boost libido, as they shape the individual's openness to sexual experiences and willingness to engage intimately with a partner.

Moreover, the role of sensory stimulation in libido can't be overstated. Sight, smell, touch, hearing, and taste all contribute to creating an atmosphere conducive to arousal. Sensory input can trigger memory and anticipation, fueling the passion that underlies sexual desire. Each sensory experience can act as a powerful catalyst in creating a mood for intimacy, making the environment an essential player in fostering libido.

Environmental and relational factors also sway libido. The stability and satisfaction of a relationship can either boost or hinder desire. Trust and emotional connection provide a fertile ground for sexual expression, while unresolved conflicts or emotional distance can act as inhibitors. The emotional safety and trust between partners facilitate vulnerability, which is paramount for a vibrant and healthy sexual connection.

Age and life stages play a critical role in libido's ebbs and flows. As individuals progress through different phases of life, changes in hormonal profiles, health conditions, and life stressors can affect sexual desire. For instance, the libido often peaks in young adults and may fluctuate during child-rearing years due to fatigue or stress. Later in life, it can be influenced by health conditions or changes in relationship dynamics.

Understanding the science behind libido involves acknowledging its inherently dynamic nature. By recognizing that desire is not static and may vary over time due to physiological, psychological, and external factors, individuals can approach their own experiences with compassion and flexibility. Being informed enables proactive steps in enhancing libido, ultimately fostering deeper connections and more fulfilling intimate relationships.

In conclusion, libido is a complex and ever-evolving phenomenon, rooted deeply in a blend of hormonal, neural, psychological, and environmental factors. By understanding these intricate workings, individuals and couples can better navigate the challenges and embrace the pleasures that desire brings. This journey of understanding can lead to an enriched sense of self and partnership, where passion is not merely a spontaneous occurrence but a cultivated and cherished bond.

Myths and Facts About Desire

Desire often finds itself at the crossroads of myth and reality, woven into the complex tapestry of human passion and intimacy. Many of us navigate our own desires with a mixture of curiosity, doubt, and anticipation. Myths about desire can obscure our understanding, keeping vital truths hidden in shadows and perpetuating misconceptions that affect our relationships.

One prevalent myth is the belief that desire is purely physical—an instinctual urge disconnected from emotional and psychological components. While physical attraction and hormones undeniably play roles in desire, it is incomplete to isolate them from emotional factors such as connection, trust, and mutual understanding with a partner. Desire is a multifaceted experience, not just a surge of hormones.

Another common misconception is that desire ought to be spontaneous and natural at all times. Movies and cultural narratives often depict desire as an ever-present, unyielding force. Yet, in reality, this is seldom the case. Desire ebbs and flows based on various life circumstances, including stress levels, life changes, and relationship dynamics. Accepting this variability allows individuals to approach their intimate lives with patience and compassion.

There's also the myth that once lost, desire is irretrievable, like a ship that's sailed never to return. This misconception can discourage individuals or couples during times when passion wanes. The truth is, desire can be rekindled. It requires intentional effort, understanding, communication, and sometimes a little help from outside sources, such as therapy or couples' workshops.

Moreover, some believe that high levels of desire correlate directly with love or relationship satisfaction. This assumption can lead to undue pressure or self-doubt, especially if one's desire naturally fluctuates. In fact, every person has a unique libido shaped by multiple factors, and variations in desire do not inherently imply dissatisfaction or lack of love.

There's an inaccurate belief that age inevitably dampens all desires. It's true that hormonal changes can influence desire as one ages, but the link between age and desire is not absolute. Many people find that their desires evolve, becoming richer and more nuanced with time and experience. Age can bring a greater understanding of one's own needs and the confidence to express them.

On the flip side, many believe that youth comes with an untamed libido that is impossible to control or understand—a misconception that can foster unrealistic expectations about sex and intimacy in young adults. Education and understanding can lead to more fulfilling and healthy intimate lives, where desire is not left unchecked but channeled through wisdom and mutual respect.

The roles of mental health, stress, and emotional well-being are often overlooked when considering desire. Many myths imply that mental well-being and desire operate independently when, in fact, they are intricately connected. Stress, anxiety, depression, and other mental health challenges can significantly impact one's libido, often requiring thoughtful attention and care to manage.

Lastly, a myth persists that discussing or seeking help for issues with desire is shameful or unnecessary, fostering a silence that stifles growth and understanding. In contrast, openly addressing these issues—either through conversation with a partner, seeking professional guidance, or exploring resources—can profoundly benefit one's intimate and emotional well-being.

Learning to distinguish myths from reality empowers individuals and couples to navigate their sexual lives with clarity and intention. Recognizing the holistic nature of desire, including its psychological, emotional, and physical underpinnings, enables us to approach intimacy with openness and understanding. We have the opportunity to explore, redefine, and enrich our desires, allowing them to mature alongside us as we grow in our relationships.

Chapter 2:
Communication and Connection

At the heart of any intimate relationship lies the vibrant dance of communication and connection, where words and gestures intertwine to create an unspoken bond. This chapter explores the profound impact of open dialogue, where sharing dreams, fears, and desires becomes the cornerstone of mutual understanding. We delve into techniques for effective communication, emphasizing the importance of active listening and the subtle art of non-verbal cues. These elements form the delicate threads that strengthen intimacy, allowing couples to navigate through challenges with grace and deepen their emotional ties. Imagine conversations as the soulful melody that accompanies the dance, guiding partners towards a more fulfilling and passionate connection. By cultivating this harmonious exchange, lovers can rediscover the thrill of desire and the comfort of a shared journey, building bridges to a more enriched and blissful relationship.

The Importance of Open Dialogue

Open dialogue is the cornerstone of any successful and intimate relationship. It's the bridge that connects two individuals, allowing for a shared understanding and mutual growth. In romantic partnerships, the freedom to express one's thoughts and feelings is paramount. When couples engage in honest communication, they pave the way for deeper connections and enhance their overall intimacy. It's not just about talking; it's about truly listening and responding with empathy and understanding.

Engaging in open dialogue involves more than just words. It requires vulnerability, courage, and sometimes confronting uncomfortable truths about ourselves and our relationships. This form of communication creates a safe space where both partners feel heard and valued. It's about breaking down barriers and building trust, which in turn can significantly enhance libido and desire. When partners feel emotionally connected, they are more likely to feel physically connected as well.

However, achieving open dialogue can be challenging. Many of us carry fears of judgment or rejection, which can inhibit our willingness to share our deepest desires and needs. To overcome these fears, it's essential to cultivate a culture of openness within the relationship. This involves establishing ground rules for communication such as listening without interrupting, expressing appreciation, and showing empathy. By doing so, partners can create an environment where dialogue flows naturally and effortlessly.

One technique to foster open dialogue is regular check-ins. Setting aside dedicated time to discuss feelings, experiences, and desires can be incredibly beneficial. These moments of connection allow partners to reflect on what is working well and what might need attention. These check-ins also provide an opportunity to express gratitude and reinforce positive behavior in the relationship, strengthening the bond over time.

Open dialogue isn't just about addressing challenges; it's also about celebrating successes and sharing joy. Expressing appreciation and acknowledging each other's efforts can build a strong foundation of positive reinforcement. This practice not only increases relationship satisfaction but also enhances attraction and desire. Partners who feel appreciated are more likely to engage in intimate acts, reinforcing the cycle of connection and desire.

Non-verbal communication plays a significant role in open dialogue. A simple touch, a warm glance, or a genuine smile can convey messages that words sometimes cannot. By being mindful of these cues, couples can deepen their understanding of each other's needs and desires, often sparking increased intimacy and excitement. Such non-verbal interactions can reaffirm the verbal commitments made during open dialogues.

Creating an atmosphere conducive to open dialogue also involves being mindful of external factors. Stress, work pressures, and personal challenges can all impact one's ability to communicate effectively. Recognizing these distractions and addressing them can prevent misunderstandings and miscommunication. This awareness helps couples stay connected and focused on nurturing their relationship, even amid life's inevitable ups and downs.

Barrier-free communication allows couples to explore and articulate their sexual needs and preferences openly. Discussing topics such as fantasies, boundaries, and experiences can demystify and destigmatize these conversations, making them a natural part of the relationship dialogue. This openness can lead to exciting discoveries and shared experiences that reignite passion and enhance both partners' satisfaction.

There is immeasurable power in expressing oneself authentically without fear of reproach. This authenticity can be transformative, leading to a partnership that thrives on mutual respect and a profound understanding of one another. It is through open dialogue that couples can reveal their authentic selves and cultivate an environment where both feel safe and cherished. In this space, intimacy flourishes naturally.

It's important to recognize that open dialogue is a dynamic process. As relationships evolve, so will the conversations within them. Being open to this fluidity and willing to adapt can help partners maintain a strong connection over time. Flexibility in communication allows couples to navigate changes and challenges more effectively, staying grounded in their shared commitment to each other.

In summary, open dialogue is a deliberate practice that requires intention, patience, and support from both partners. It's a continuous journey of learning and growth, offering endless opportunities to deepen intimacy and connection. By embracing open dialogue, couples can enhance their emotional and physical connection, leading to a more fulfilling and passionate relationship.

As you embark on your journey of cultivating open dialogue, remember that every conversation is a building block towards a more profound and meaningful partnership. The ability to communicate honestly and empathetically is one of the greatest gifts you can give to your relationship. It's an investment in yourself, your partner, and the shared love that binds you.

Techniques for Effective Communication

Nurturing a dynamic intimate connection often hinges on our ability to communicate effectively. While words are a fundamental conduit, effective communication transcends mere conversation. It's about embracing vulnerability and honesty in each interaction, allowing space for both partners to express desires and fears without judgment. This requires a harmonious blend of verbal and non-verbal cues, reflecting empathy and understanding in every gesture and phrase. To truly connect, partners must actively listen, not just with their ears but with their hearts, creating a safe environment where each can be genuinely heard and valued. As you expand these skills, you'll find they act as a cornerstone not just for enhancing libido but also for deepening the emotional intimacy that enriches every layer of your relationship.

Active Listening in Relationships is an unsung hero in the symphony of effective communication. At its core, active listening goes beyond merely hearing the words spoken by a partner—it's an immersive practice that can turn a mundane exchange into a deeply connecting experience. In relationships, it's a bridge that can span the potential divide between two people, fostering intimacy, understanding, and a renewed sense of harmony. Imagine conversations where both partners feel truly heard and understood, where the art of listening becomes as intoxicating as the allure of desire itself.

Let's paint a picture for a moment: you're sitting across from your partner, eyes locked in a dance of mutual interest. You lean in slightly, making it clear that every word they speak is a gift, prioritizing the moment you're sharing over the buzz of a phone or the distractions of the day. Your responses, instead of being immediate, are thoughtful, acknowledging not just what was said, but what's unsaid—the hopes, fears, and dreams woven into the fabric of their words. This is active listening in its purest form.

Active listening can transform relationships by validating the speaker and inviting a deeper exploration of their thoughts and emotions. For many, the daily grind and life's pressures can create a cloud of disconnection. We often listen to respond rather than to understand, leading to miscommunication and hurt feelings. But embracing active listening shifts the focus from our immediate reactions to our partner's inner world, fostering a sense of safety and trust.

To truly commit to active listening, one must engage both with their heart and mind. This means being attuned to your partner's verbal and non-verbal cues. It's about catching the slight change in their tone, noticing the pauses that signal reflection, and understanding the emotions that aren't always articulated. Such mindfulness can enrich conversations, helping partners feel more secure in sharing their authentic selves.

In the tapestry of communication, feedback plays a pivotal role. Active listening isn't passive; it involves providing authentic, empathetic responses that convey support and understanding. Techniques such as paraphrasing—repeating what your partner has said in your own words—can clarify and affirm that you've grasped the essence of their message. Imagine a moment of vulnerability where your partner expresses a concern, and you respond with "What I'm hearing is that you're feeling overwhelmed by everything right now. Is that right?" This simple act acknowledges their feelings and opens the door for further conversation and emotional connection.

Moreover, questions are an essential tool in the active listener's toolbox—open-ended inquiries that invite elaboration and continued dialogue, avoiding the conversational dead ends that 'yes' or 'no' questions often impose. Asking questions like "How did that make you feel?" or "What do you think we can do to make things better?" demonstrates a genuine desire to delve deeper, uncovering layers that might otherwise remain buried.

Active listening also involves suspension of judgment. At times, preconceived notions or past experiences may color our perception of what's being said. In those moments, it's crucial to approach each interaction with an open heart and mind, viewing our partner's words as a snapshot of their current reality rather than a trigger for past grievances. This neutral, patient stance allows us to gather information that clarifies the situation rather than clouding it with bias.

Reflection is another component of active listening that strengthens intimacy. By taking time after a conversation to ponder what was discussed and how it impacts your relationship, you can gain insights into patterns or concerns that might benefit from attention. This kind of thoughtful reflection is a pathway to growth, offering an opportunity to nurture the relationship with intention and care.

Active listening isn't perfect every time. We all have moments where stress or external distractions make it challenging to be fully present. What's important is the commitment to returning to this practice, acknowledging where improvements can be made, and striving to enhance conversations in the future. Even a simple acknowledgment like, "I wasn't fully present just now, but I'd love to hear more when you're ready," can be a healing balm for any missteps along the way.

The transformative power of active listening can't be overstated. It can bridge gaps, mend rifts, and solidify the foundation upon which intimacy is built. Through these acts of attentive engagement, partners feel cherished and heard, nurturing a cycle of trust and openness that enhances their intimate connection. By embracing this technique, relationships can flourish, breathing new life into the dance of desire and connection they share.

Non-Verbal Communication is a powerful language in its own right, often speaking volumes without uttering a single word. In the realm of intimate relationships, where emotions run deep and connections are paramount, understanding and mastering non-verbal cues can be transformative. Everyday gestures, expressions, and silent exchanges carry meanings that convey trust, empathy, and understanding, allowing partners to connect on a profound level.

In an intimate relationship setting, non-verbal communication can often transcend the spoken word, acting as a bridge to deeper understanding and connection. A gentle touch, a prolonged gaze, or a subtle facial expression can carry messages that words struggle to capture. Imagine the comfort of a reassuring nod or the warmth of a genuine smile; these small acts are loaded with significance, capable of affirming, comforting, and sometimes, healing. Partners who learn to read and reciprocate these cues often find themselves navigating the complexities of intimacy with greater ease.

It's crucial to recognize the role of body language in expressing desire and creating a romantic atmosphere. Body language can ignite passion and melt away hesitation, as the signals exchanged silently can fuel the chemistry between lovers. Whether it's the gentle brush of hands or the way one's body naturally leans toward the other, these gestures can express longing and eagerness, setting the stage for deeper emotional and physical connections. Non-verbal cues are not just ancillary to spoken language; they are sometimes even more reliable indicators of true feelings.

Moreover, the power of eye contact cannot be overstated. It is often said that the eyes are the windows to the soul, and in the context of relationships, this becomes especially true. A partner who maintains eye contact while listening shows attentiveness and interest, signaling that they value what is being shared. On the other hand, a gentle, lingering gaze can communicate love and admiration, adding layers of depth to romantic interaction. Eye contact builds intimacy, enhances trust, and can rekindle passion when words may seem inadequate.

Facial expressions serve as another potent component of non-verbal communication. The human face is capable of an incredible range of emotions, from joy to sadness, surprise to assurance. When partners become adept at reading each other's facial expressions, they can respond more sensitively to unspoken needs, creating a sense of being understood without delving into complicated conversations. This skill fosters a nurturing environment where emotional authenticity thrives, allowing couples to be genuinely vulnerable with one another.

While gestures like hand-holding or caresses are common forms of physical connection, their significance is often underestimated. These actions can convey a sense of safety and belongingness, reassuring a partner of one's commitment and affection. Tender touch releases oxytocin, often referred to as the 'love hormone,' which strengthens bonds and promotes emotional warmth. The simplicity of holding hands can silently articulate a promise of togetherness, especially during challenging times, reinforcing a sense of love and unity.

The role of space and proximity in non-verbal communication is equally important. The physical space or distance a person maintains can tell a lot about their comfort, interest, and emotional state. In intimate relationships, closeness tends to symbolize trust and affection. Engaging in activities that naturally bring partners closer, like dancing or cuddling, takes advantage of this aspect of non-verbal communication, encouraging connection through shared physical space and mutual enjoyment.

Non-verbal communication also plays a significant role in resolving conflicts and misunderstandings. When words become sharp and tense, the calming presence of a loving embrace or a gentle touch can de-escalate tensions, offering solace and compassion when dialogue falters. Partners who use non-verbal signals effectively during disagreements often find resolutions faster, as these gestures remind each other of the underlying love and respect that outlasts any single argument.

Furthermore, shared routines and rituals serve as foundational pillars for enduring relationships, communicated through habitual non-verbal acts. Whether it's a morning routine of brewing coffee for one another or a nightly ritual of reflecting on the day's highlights, these routines convey commitment and love through consistent care, emphasizing shared experiences and highlighting the nuances of silent communication.

It's important for couples to grow their awareness and understanding of non-verbal signals, paving a path to greater intimacy and harmony. This necessitates an openness to learning and adapting, paying close attention to the silent messages exchanged daily. By consciously embracing this form of communication, partners can enrich their relationship, bridging any gaps that words might leave open. Clear communication becomes multilayered and nuanced, rooted both in the gestures shared and in the understanding they foster.

Encouraging genuine non-verbal interactions can elevate sexual experiences as well, as partners become more attuned to each other's rhythms and desires. Silent pauses and mutual breaths can set the tone, creating a synchrony that elevates physical connections beyond mere act—the emotional resonance is intensified, matching the shared physicality with an emotional cadence that vibrates through partners' shared experiences.

Overall, the art of non-verbal communication in intimacy is about creating a love language that's implicitly understood, deepening the symbiosis between partners. Encouraging each other's growth in this language transforms it from subtle communication to a profound expression of love. As partners learn to navigate this spectrum of communication, they unlock new dimensions of closeness, building a robust foundation of empathy, passion, and understanding. Such mastery ensures that the relationship continues to thrive, offering a fertile ground for intimacy to flourish, for dreams to be shared, and for a love that's palpable, yet serenely spoken without uttering a word.

Chapter 3:
Physical Fitness and Libido

In the vibrant dance of intimacy and connection, physical fitness emerges as a vital partner, enlivening the rhythm of desire and enriching the tapestry of love. Engaging in regular exercise not only sculpts the body but also harmonizes the intricate symphony of hormones that drive libido. As endorphins surge and blood circulation improves, a renewed vitality breathes life into both passion and performance, fostering a deeper connection with your partner. Explore the transformative power of movement, recognizing how each heartbeat during cardiovascular activities and every strengthening stance in resistance training builds more than muscle—it fortifies the bridge between physical wellness and heightened erotic energy. Embrace the invigorating journey of fitness as a means of celebrating and amplifying your intimate bonds, unleashing a newfound desire that speaks to the heart's yearning for closeness and the soul's quest for connection.

Exercise and Hormone Balance

In the delicate dance of human desire, hormones play the role of an orchestra conductor, orchestrating the symphony of feelings and libido. Exercise, like a skillful musician, can play its part in tuning this orchestra to achieve harmony. When it comes to balancing hormones, the benefits of regular physical activity extend far beyond the familiar realms of weight management or cardiovascular health—they reach into the intricate web of hormonal balance that fuels our sexual desire and intimacy.

In essence, our bodies are dynamic systems responding to stimuli in complex ways, and exercise proves to be a compelling input. It affects the levels of various hormones such as testosterone, estrogen, cortisol, and endorphins, all of which are significant players in the libido landscape. Testosterone, often heralded as the "hormone of desire," is crucial for both men and women. While men naturally have higher levels, it's significant in women, too; both genders see a benefit in libido from exercise-induced increases.

Consider a brisk 30-minute run. As you lace up, your body gears up for action, releasing endorphins that boost your mood and reduce stress. That runner's high isn't just a metaphor; it's a tangible shift in hormonal balance, with endorphins acting like tiny neurotransmitter heroes, battling stress and anxiety that often act as barriers to libido. These neurochemicals foster feelings of euphoria and relaxation, making you more receptive to intimacy.

Strength training adds another layer to this hormonal interplay. When you lift weights or engage in resistance training, you're not just sculpting muscles—you're nudging your body into releasing more testosterone. The increased levels can enhance libido by reviving the vigor and passion that might have waned under modern life's stressors. Focusing on major muscle groups like the legs, chest, and back can lead to a significant increase in testosterone production, acting as nature's aphrodisiac.

Yet, it's not just about testosterone. Estrogen, often spotlighted for its role in reproductive health in women, also plays an essential part in libido for both sexes. Regular physical activity helps maintain optimal levels of estrogen, which can fluctuate due to stress or aging. For women, exercise helps alleviate symptoms of menopause by balancing estrogen levels, which can consequently boost libido. Meanwhile, for men, proper estrogen balance ensures healthy sexual functionality.

Moreover, the role of exercise in reducing cortisol, the infamous "stress hormone," cannot be overlooked. Even the most ardent romantic interludes can be hampered by elevated cortisol, which erodes libido. Regular activities like yoga or tai chi harmonize the body's stress responses, lowering cortisol levels and creating an environment where desire can flourish. This impact extends beyond a single workout session, leading to long-term improvements in how our bodies handle stress.

Beyond these direct hormonal effects, exercise contributes to better sleep and mood, indirectly boosting libido. A body that is rested and rejuvenated is more likely to respond to the beckon of romantic desires. Improved sleep patterns foster a positive feedback loop, leading to better hormone regulation—a cycle that healthily perpetuates itself.

Consider the indirect yet powerful impact of body confidence. Exercise helps many individuals feel more comfortable in their skin, boosting self-esteem and positively impacting libido. Feeling attractive and desirable to oneself can be profoundly empowering, building the foundation for more authentic and fulfilling intimate experiences. When you feel confident about the body you inhabit, it reflects in your openness to sharing that body with someone else.

The social aspect of exercise shouldn't be underestimated either. Joining a class, whether it's spinning, dancing, or crossfit, can offer communal support and motivation, thereby enhancing emotional well-being. Interactions with others who share similar fitness goals can cultivate a sense of belonging and happiness, indirectly nurturing a more robust libido.

One might think of exercising as a daily ritual rather than a chore. In doing so, it becomes interwoven with our intrinsic routines, subtly but powerfully aligning hormones for optimal balance. Establishing a consistent routine of physical activity aligns well with maintaining a steady hormonal equilibrium, and the benefits compound over time.

While integrating physical fitness into your lifestyle for libido enhancement, it's essential to honor your body's uniqueness. Each of us responds differently due to genetics, current health conditions, and lifestyle factors. Thus, a personalized approach to exercise will be more effective in finding that perfect hormonal homeostasis.

As you embark on this journey, remember that the rewards of exercise are not just visible in physical transformations; they resonate deeply in the undercurrents of your body's biochemistry. By embracing exercise as a tool to fine-tune hormone balance, you're setting the stage for an enriched intimate life, where both passion and connection can flourish alongside the physiological benefits that endure.

Types of Exercises to Boost Desire

In the realm of physical fitness and its profound connection to libido, selecting the right types of exercises can serve as a powerful catalyst for enhancing desire. Engaging in cardiovascular training, such as brisk walking, swimming, or cycling, increases heart rate and promotes better blood flow, which is vital for sexual health. On the other hand, strength training, involving activities like weightlifting or bodyweight exercises, contributes to hormone balance by boosting testosterone levels, which play a critical role in sexual desire for all genders. These exercises not only sculpt the body but also enhance confidence, which is inherently attractive and can lead to a more fulfilling romantic experience. By weaving exercise into your routine, you're not just nurturing your physical well-being, but also stoking the embers of passion and intimacy, paving the way for a thriving connection with your partner.

Cardiovascular Training enhances not just the heart's capacity to support life's demands, but it also fuels the very essence of desire and passion. When blood flows with ease, energized by a healthy heart, it benefits not only the body's core but also the intimacy shared between partners. Regular cardiovascular exercise isn't just a means of staying fit; it's a potent tool for amplifying libido, breathing life into passion that might be lying dormant.

Consider the rhythm of a brisk walk, the challenge of a cycling session, or the exhilaration of a swim. These activities heighten heart rate and circulation, delivering oxygen-rich blood throughout the body. This surge in blood flow nurtures all organs, including those pivotal in sexual function. By improving circulation, cardiovascular training ensures that bodily systems work harmoniously, leading to improved sexual arousal and orgasmic response times.

Moreover, the biochemical cascade triggered by cardiovascular training plays a noteworthy role in stoking the fires of desire. Exercise is known to reduce stress hormones like cortisol while simultaneously boosting endorphins—those "feel-good" neurotransmitters that elevate mood and create a sense of well-being. An uplifted mood naturally feeds into enhanced body confidence, reducing anxiety around intimacy. This mental uplift is mirrored by the increase in vital hormones, such as testosterone and estrogen, which are crucial in sexual health and desire. Research continually shows that these hormonal benefits from regular cardiovascular exercise lay the groundwork for increased libido.

The variety in cardiovascular training options offers a dynamic approach suited to individual preferences and lifestyles. From jogging through scenic trails to heart-pounding dance classes, the diversity of choices empowers individuals or couples to find what best fits their routines and goals. Engaging in such activities together can transform workout time into a bonding experience that fosters emotional and physical connections. Sharing laughter and encouragement during a spirited game of tennis or pushing each other's limits during a hike can nurture the relationship, making mutual fitness goals an intimate journey.

For those just beginning their cardiovascular journey, it's about setting realistic, enjoyable goals. Start small, perhaps with a few minutes of walking supplemented with bursts of higher intensity, and gradually build up as comfort allows. Incorporate activities that spark joy and encourage regularity rather than obligation. Combining these exercises with mindfulness, such as focusing on breath and bodily sensations, transforms mundane routine into enriching experiences that build anticipation and excitement for shared moments.

The transformative nature of cardiovascular training doesn't stop at the physiological. When two people engage in regular cardiovascular exercise, there is an undeniable boost to their collective confidence in and out of the bedroom. Embarking on this journey encourages mutual growth and shared achievements that can affirm each partner's value beyond physical appearance—an important factor in sustaining passion. By prioritizing health, couples inadvertently demonstrate care for one another, reinforcing emotional bonds and trust.

Additionally, beyond the physical and emotional spheres, there lies a cerebral aspect. Cardiovascular exercise can enhance cognitive function, leading to improved mood regulation and increased empathy—both critical components in maintaining a healthy balance in relationships. With enhanced mental acuity, partners become better equipped to communicate effectively and to understand each other's needs, further elevating their sexual and emotional connection.

As with any lifestyle modification, the key is consistency. Adopting cardiovascular training into one's routine is a declaration of commitment—both to personal health and to the shared journey of intimacy with a partner. This commitment yields a blueprint for living life with vibrancy and passion, ensuring that energies devoted to physical fitness are rewarded not just with health, but with deeper intimacy and renewed desire.

To truly unlock its potential, it helps to consider what cardiovascular training reflects in the broader context of love and sexuality—movement, vitality, and union. In many ways, cardio is a mirror of what lies at the core of healthy desire: an acknowledgment of ebb and flow, of sustained effort interspersed with intense bursts of love and passion.

Ultimately, cardiovascular training as part of a routine to boost libido is a profound declaration of valuing oneself and one's partner. It carries with it an inspiring message—one of hope and rejuvenation. By engaging in these active choices, partners honor and nourish the body and soul in equal measure, laying the groundwork not just for physical intimacy but for a heartfelt connection—a celebration of both love and life, indulged in with openness and joy.

Strength Training is not just about building muscle and sculpting your body; it's a powerful tool in nurturing a thriving libido. Within the context of physical fitness and its impact on desire, strength training plays an influential role in boosting hormone production, particularly testosterone, which is a key player in sexual arousal for both men and women. But how does lifting weights translate into more passion in the bedroom? The answer lies in both physiological transformations and mental empowerment.

Strength training stimulates the release of endorphins, those magical neurotransmitters that reduce stress and promote a sense of well-being and relaxation. In today's fast-paced world, stress often serves as a significant libido killer. By incorporating regular strength training sessions into your routine, you pave the way for diminishing stress and enhancing your intimate life. It's like having a natural antidote to anxiety, vastly improving the atmosphere in which desire can flourish.

Moreover, this form of exercise develops confidence, which is intrinsically linked to enhanced desire. As muscles grow and you achieve personal fitness milestones, a sense of accomplishment blossoms. This feeling of self-assuredness doesn't just linger in the gym but transcends into other areas of life, including your intimate interactions. Confidence fosters an open, adventurous spirit, making you more receptive to exploring new sensuous experiences with your partner.

Physiologically, strength training boosts circulation, which is vital for sexual health. Improved blood flow means increased oxygen to muscles and organs, including those involved in sexual arousal. A robust circulatory system supports the body's capacity to respond to physical and environmental cues, thus potentially leading to heightened sexual experiences. It translates to an enhanced ability to engage in and maintain desire, making those shared moments even more exhilarating.

And let's not forget the emotional aspects. Strength training encourages goal-setting, discipline, and perseverance. These attributes carry over into the relationship sphere, promoting a mutual journey of support and growth. When partners embark on a fitness journey together, it fosters unity and understanding, laying a strong foundation for an intimate and fulfilling relationship. Imagine the shared joy of overcoming a challenging workout session and the sense of achievement that bonds you even closer.

Let's delve into a typical workout regimen suitable for boosting libido through strength training. Consider compound exercises like squats, deadlifts, and bench presses, which engage multiple muscle groups and maximize hormonal response. These movements are highly effective at increasing the natural production of testosterone and growth hormone, essential for both muscle and libido enhancement. Start with lower weights to perfect form, gradually increasing as you gain strength.

For those unfamiliar with strength training or hesitant to hit the gym, home-based bodyweight exercises can also be effective. Exercises such as push-ups, lunges, and planks not only enhance muscular strength but also improve core stability and balance, which can lead to increased confidence during intimate moments. A simple at-home circuit could consist of three sets of 10-15 repetitions of each exercise, performed thrice weekly.

Combining strength training with other types of exercise, such as cardiovascular activities and stretching, rounds out a balanced fitness program that supports overall health and vitality. Each type of physical activity contributes uniquely, creating a harmonious environment for a vibrant libido. The synergy between elevated heart health from cardio, muscle growth from strength training, and flexibility from stretching prepares the body for both daily challenges and delightful intimate encounters.

Consistency is crucial. Establish a routine that fits seamlessly into your weekly schedule. This integration ensures long-term benefits, making strength training a sustainable part of your lifestyle rather than a short-term endeavor. As your physical fitness evolves, so will your capacity for desire, creating a perpetual cycle of positive reinforcement.

Moreover, strength training invites a deeper understanding and appreciation of your own body. Awareness of physical capabilities and boundaries enhances body positivity, a factor often overlooked but critical in sexual well-being. When you respect and admire your body's achievements, you bring a kind of magnetism into intimate situations that's both empowering and attractive to your partner.

Incorporate mindfulness into your training sessions. Tune into your body's movements, focusing on the sensations and connecting with each lift and breath. This practice enhances your mind-body connection, a bridge that fortifies the overlap between physicality and sensual consciousness. It brings the mental presence necessary to fully enjoy and cherish intimate moments, making each encounter unforgettable.

There's an inherent romance in the discipline of strength training, a rhythm that parallels the dance of desire. As with any romance, cultivation is key. Each training session is an invitation to deepen your relationship with your body, to understand its desires and fulfill them. The synergy found in a well-tuned physique often translates into a vibrant, energetic sexual appetite.

As you embrace the power of strength training, remember it's not just a solitary pursuit but a shared journey. Encouraging your partner to join can amplify the benefits, leading to a mutual exploration of strength, health, and intimacy. Together, you're not just building physical resilience but also crafting a shared life rich in passion and connection.

Chapter 4:
Nutrition and Libido

In this chapter, we delve into the fascinating interplay between nutrition and libido, offering insights that elevate both your dietary habits and your intimate life. The foods we consume play a pivotal role in fueling our passions and desires. Nutrient-rich foods like dark chocolate, avocados, and oysters have long been celebrated for their aphrodisiac properties, providing a tantalizing boost to your libido. Meanwhile, supplements containing essential vitamins and minerals, such as zinc and vitamin B6, can support hormonal balance and reproductive health. Incorporating these into your routine not only nurtures your physical health but also fosters a deeper emotional and romantic connection with your partner. As you explore dietary choices that enhance vitality, you begin a journey towards a more fulfilling and intimate relationship, powered by the simple yet profound influence of nutrition.

Foods That Enhance Desire

Nutrition has a profound impact on many aspects of our well-being, including the intricate dance of desire. While a healthy libido is influenced by a multitude of factors, the foods we choose can significantly contribute to enhancing our sexual vitality. Imagine a dining experience where each bite brings you closer to your loved one, not only in proximity but in passion as well. Certain foods have been celebrated, not only in modern times but across centuries and cultures, as natural aphrodisiacs. These are the ingredients that whisper secrets of increased blood flow, hormone balance, and improved mood—all crucial elements for a thriving libido.

Dark chocolate is often hailed as a cupid among foods, renowned for its ability to ignite sparks of desire. Rich in flavonoids, dark chocolate can help to increase blood circulation and lower stress levels, two pivotal aspects of sexual health. The mere taste and texture might stir feelings of luxury and indulgence, creating a sensory experience that pairs delightfully with candlelit moments and whispered sentiments. But more than just a mood setter, the phenylethylamine in chocolate encourages the release of endorphins, our body's own "feel-good" chemicals.

Consider, too, the subtle allure of oysters. Not only are they symbols of sophisticated indulgence, but they also pack a punch with their high zinc content. Zinc is crucial for the production of testosterone, the hormone that fuels libido in both men and women. While the texture and taste of oysters might not appeal to everyone, they stand as a testament to the power of food in enhancing desire, especially when enjoyed fresh with a squeeze of lemon and a dash of passionate intent.

Sometimes, the way to desire is through the heart of fruits and vegetables. Avocados, with their creamy texture and rich nutrient profile, are named the "fruit of the Gods" for a reason. They are packed with vitamin B6, which is essential for the production of male hormones, and potassium, which helps regulate the thyroid gland in females. Nutrients from avocados support not just physical health, but also the energy and endurance needed for intimate encounters.

When you delve into the world of spices, you uncover treasures like saffron. A single thread embodies centuries of use as an aphrodisiac, with studies suggesting it improves sexual behavior and satisfaction. Saffron adds a vibrant golden hue to dishes but, more importantly, inspires golden moments of connection with its subtle scent and flavor. Similarly, the sultry allure of cinnamon invigorates the senses and stimulates blood circulation, adding warmth to the body both inside and out.

For those looking for a truly exotic twist, figs and pomegranates have long been associated with love and fertility. Figs, with their delicate and sweet flesh, are ripe with iron and magnesium, ensuring balanced energy levels and muscular health, which can be vital in moments of passion. Pomegranates, on the other hand, are not only visually beautiful but were revered in ancient cultures for their potential to enhance fertility and increase sexual potency with their abundance of antioxidants.

Nutty delights like almonds and walnuts offer their own benefits. Rich in omega-3 fatty acids and vitamin E, these nuts regulate hormones and provide ample energy, making them a nourishing partner to a passionate partnership. By promoting heart health and circulation, the humble almond becomes an ally in extending the pleasures of intimacy.

Then there are those fiery red wonders, chili peppers. These add more than just heat to your dishes; they stimulate endorphins and increase your heart rate, mimicking the natural responses of arousal. The vibrant spice is a testament to the thrill of experiencing shared moments of fiery excitement and emotional connection.

While individual preferences and dietary needs vary, the shared experience of enjoying a meal rich with aphrodisiac properties can be a loving gesture in itself. The act of choosing ingredients thoughtfully, creating dishes with care, and savoring them together fosters a sense of connection and anticipation. Ultimately, the key is to harness these foods as part of an overall lifestyle that supports not only a healthy libido but a joyful, intimate relationship.

Incorporating these foods into your diet, with love and creativity, can help pave the way to a more vibrant intimate life. But remember, while they may enhance desire, it is the shared experiences and mutual effort between partners that truly light the flame of passion. Whether paired with a sweet serenade or a quiet evening together, these foods might just be the gentle nudge that turns desire into an action, and moments into treasured memories.

The Role of Supplements

When it comes to enhancing libido through nutrition, supplements can play a significant part in bridging any gaps your diet might have left open. They can offer a potent blend of essential vitamins, minerals, and herbal remedies known to support sexual health and increase desire. For instance, supplements like L-arginine, zinc, and ginseng have been studied for their potential to boost blood flow and hormonal balance, which are crucial for a vibrant sexual appetite. However, while supplements can be beneficial, they work best in harmony with a well-rounded diet and a healthy lifestyle. It's always wise to consult with a healthcare professional before starting any supplement regimen to ensure they complement your unique nutritional needs and health goals. By thoughtfully incorporating these aids, you are taking deliberate steps towards invigorating your libido, thus nurturing the intimate connection you share with your partner.

Essential Vitamins and Minerals play a vital role in enhancing libido, acting as fundamental components that fuel our bodies and, by extension, our desires. These micronutrients serve as the catalysts for numerous biochemical reactions, which can help in maintaining a healthy sexual desire. Nutritionally vibrant diets provide these critical elements, but sometimes, a hectic lifestyle or dietary restrictions may lead us to consider supplements.

Vitamins and minerals are not just essential for basic health; they directly affect your libido and overall sexual well-being. Let's begin with vitamin D, a powerful mood stabilizer and immune booster that holds promise beyond its conventional roles. Not only does vitamin D help in maintaining bone health, but it's also pivotal for testosterone production. Low levels of this vitamin can lead to decreased testosterone in men, which might impact sexual drive and performance.

Another essential vitamin is B-complex, a group of eight different vitamins that collectively work to elevate energy levels and improve circulation. Vitamin B6, in particular, is indispensable as it helps balance sex hormones, which are critical for libido. In women, vitamin B6 can help regulate the levels of estrogen and progesterone, two hormones vital for sexual health.

Then we have Vitamin E, often referred to as the "sex vitamin." Its power lies in its antioxidant properties, which support blood flow and offer protection against oxidative stress. Vitamin E assists in maintaining healthy skin and blood vessels, elements essential for sexual arousal and function. Regular intake through diet or supplements can rejuvenate your sense of intimacy by enhancing circulation and stamina.

The mineral zinc is often underrated but holds immense power in fueling desire and arousal. Zinc is crucial in the production of testosterone, and its deficiency can manifest as reduced libido. Ensuring an adequate intake of zinc can improve both the quality of sperm and overall sexual functionality in men. How much do you need? It's often as simple as having more seeds, nuts, or perhaps a high-quality supplement if your diet falls short.

Magnesium offers another layer of support, especially for those dealing with stress and fatigue, two notorious libido inhibitors. Taking magnesium can assist in relaxing your muscles and alleviating stress, promoting a peaceful mind that's more amenable to intimacy. With its influence on muscle function and mood stabilization, this mineral is a quiet hero when it comes to enhancing your intimate moments.

Keep in mind that while these vitamins and minerals can play a significant role in boosting libido, they should be part of a balanced and whole lifestyle approach. Supplements shouldn't replace a well-rounded diet but can fill nutritional gaps. It's important to consult with healthcare providers to tailor individual needs. The right balance of vitamins and minerals can harmonize with your inner desires, helping you unlock the door to a more vibrant and fulfilling intimate life.

Herbal Remedies have long held a special place in the realm of natural health, revered for their potential to enhance not just general well-being but also specific aspects such as libido. In the intricate dance of romance and passion, where nutrition plays a pivotal role, herbs can serve as powerful allies in reinvigorating desire. Their appeal stems from centuries-old traditions combined with contemporary findings that suggest they can indeed make a meaningful difference. For those seeking to boost their intimate connections, herbal remedies offer a path that is as intriguing as it is promising.

Before diving into specific herbs, let's take a moment to understand why these remedies matter. Herbs contain bioactive compounds that can influence bodily functions, often working subtly yet effectively to address deficiencies or imbalances. They are not quick fixes but rather gentle yet consistent aids that contribute to the overall vitality of the body, including sexual health. What makes them particularly appealing is their natural origin, which aligns with those looking to avoid more synthetic options. Remember, enhancing libido is as much about nourishing the body as it is about reigniting the soul.

When considering herbal remedies, ginseng often appears at the top of the list. A well-regarded adaptogen, ginseng is famous for its ability to support energy levels and reduce stress, two factors deeply intertwined with libido. One of its key benefits is the improvement of blood flow, critical for sexual function. Ginseng's impact isn't limited to men; it can also enhance arousal and satisfaction in women, making it a versatile option for those exploring herbal paths to desire.

Moving along the garden of herbal solutions, another name that stands out is maca root. This Peruvian herb has gained popularity for its unique ability to boost stamina and endurance, features that naturally extend to enhancing libido. Not just limited to physical aspects, maca also appears to improve mood and alleviate symptoms of anxiety, indirectly benefiting one's sex drive. By fostering an inner sense of well-being and relaxation, it paves the way for more fulfilling intimate moments.

Let's not forget the aromatic and soothing qualities of lavender. Traditionally used for its calming effects, lavender's role in enhancing libido is connected to its ability to reduce anxiety and promote relaxation. The scent of lavender has been noted to increase blood flow and stimulate arousal subtly, a fact that speaks volumes about the psychological aspects of desire. By releasing the tension and creating a more conducive environment for intimacy, lavender serves as a fragrant key to unlocking closeness.

Among the more exotic options, yohimbe bark is worth mentioning. Its potency lies in its active ingredient, yohimbine, which has been shown to improve erectile function by increasing blood flow. However, yohimbe should be approached with caution due to its strong effects and potential side effects. It stands as a reminder that while herbal remedies can offer significant benefits, they must be used judiciously and often under professional guidance.

Tribulus terrestris is another herb gaining attention for its potential to boost libido. Often utilized in traditional medicine to enhance fertility and rejuvenate sexual drive, tribulus works by potentially increasing testosterone levels and improving overall vitality. Such enhancements are crucial for both physical performance and psychological readiness when it comes to intimacy. For couples seeking a more balanced and energetic interaction, tribulus offers an intriguing option to explore.

For those exploring holistic ways to enhance intimacy, ashwagandha presents a multifaceted approach. Known for its ability to improve strength, reduce stress, and increase endurance, this herb is celebrated in Ayurvedic medicine for enhancing overall quality of life, which naturally extends to sexual health. By helping to rebalance hormones and reduce cortisol levels, ashwagandha supports a more harmonious and passionate relationship.

Often overshadowed by its more well-known counterparts, fenugreek deserves a rightful place in the discussion. Particularly beneficial for women, fenugreek is believed to enhance sexual arousal and satisfaction by positively influencing hormonal balance. Men too find benefit in fenugreek's potential to improve libido and vitality. Its widespread availability and mild nature make it a popular choice for those beginning their journey into herbal remedies.

Herbal remedies, when used thoughtfully, can be an enriching addition to one's sexual wellness routine. They offer not just physical benefits but extend a sense of connection to nature, grounding individuals in a tradition that has been appreciated for generations. However, it's essential to highlight the importance of quality and sourcing when it comes to herbs. Investing in certified organic and ethically harvested options ensures you receive the most benefit without the risk of contaminants or unethical practices.

The path to enhancing libido through herbal remedies should also be coupled with an awareness of one's individual needs and reactions. Not every herb suits every person; what works wonders for one may have little effect on another. Personal experimentation, listening to your body's responses, and possibly consulting with a healthcare professional are vital steps in this journey.

Ultimately, exploring herbal remedies is about more than just boosting libido. It's an endeavor that can lead to greater self-awareness and profound intimacy. When combined with other elements like diet, communication, and emotional connection, herbs can complement the multifaceted effort to cultivate not just sexual desire, but a richer, more meaningful union with your partner.

Chapter 5:
Emotional Intimacy and Connection

Emotional intimacy forms the heart of a fulfilling relationship, cultivating a connection that goes beyond the physical and into the profound depths of trust and vulnerability. It's about forging a bond that allows couples to share their innermost thoughts and feelings, free from judgment. As we learn to open up emotionally, we pave the way for a deeper connection where empathy and support become the cornerstones of our partnership. This is not just about having someone to lean on, but also about actively listening and embracing each other's emotional worlds, thus weaving a fabric of mutual understanding and respect. Such intimacy not only rejuvenates the libido but also enriches the spirit, creating a partnership that thrives on sincerity and connection, setting the stage for more passionate and enduring love.

Building Trust and Vulnerability

Emotional intimacy serves as the core of any deeply connected relationship. It's an ever-evolving journey that requires effort, patience, and a willingness to open up to your partner. At its heart are two powerful elements: trust and vulnerability. Together, they form the bedrock of an emotional connection, fortifying the bonds of love and desire.

Trust isn't something that materializes overnight. It's a remarkable facet of human connection that grows over time, nurtured by actions, words, and consistency. Trusting someone means you feel safe and supported, and most importantly, you believe in each other's intentions. In intimate relationships, where emotions run deep and raw, trust becomes a precious currency. It's built through small, consistent gestures—keeping promises, showing up as a reliable partner, and being there when it matters most. Every act of care, every word of encouragement, slowly but surely weaves the fabric of trust stronger.

Vulnerability, on the other hand, is the willingness to be seen in all our imperfect glory. It's about letting down our shields and allowing someone to look past our defenses. In relationships, showing vulnerability means sharing thoughts, fears, dreams, and insecurities. It's trusting your partner to hold your truths gently. By being vulnerable, we allow our partners to connect with our genuine selves, fostering a deeper understanding and empathy. It's an act of courage, and this openness paves the way for authentic intimacy.

Consider vulnerability a dance—a delicate balance where giving and receiving happen in harmony. When one partner opens up, it invites the other to do the same, creating a shared experience that is both powerful and profound. This dance requires attentive listening and non-judgmental communication, where partners hold space for each other's revelations without rushing to fix or advise. Just listening can often be the most loving response.

Creating an environment where trust and vulnerability can flourish demands intentional action. It starts with everyday interactions. Words have power, and language can either build bridges or walls. Make it a practice to engage in conversations that encourage openness. Asking gentle questions about feelings, affirming each other's experiences, and practicing empathy by putting yourself in your partner's shoes can significantly bolster trust.

Boundaries also play a vital role in establishing trust and vulnerability. These invisible lines define what is acceptable and protect each partner's emotional well-being. Having honest discussions about boundaries clarifies expectations and reassures both partners that their limits are respected. This mutual respect reinforces trust and promotes an environment where vulnerability feels safe.

Interestingly, challenges and conflicts, when navigated skillfully, can provide opportunities to deepen trust. Overcoming misunderstandings or disagreements together demonstrates resilience and commitment to the relationship. It shows that even in the face of difficulties, partners are willing to stand by each other and work through issues in a constructive manner. Learning to apologize sincerely and forgive genuinely rekindles trust, proving unconditional support.

Trust is also reinforced by addressing jealousy or insecurity head on. These emotions can be tricky, but they often stem from fear or past experiences. It's crucial to have open dialogues about these feelings without judgment, exploring their roots, and addressing them with empathy and understanding. In such tender discussions, vulnerability plays a starring role, helping to dismantle walls of fear.

For partners eager to build trust and vulnerability, setting aside regular time for check-ins can be invaluable. Whether it's a cozy evening on the couch or a walk in the park, these moments of connection allow couples to express what's on their minds and hearts. It's a chance to realign and reinforce their commitment to each other, discussing anything from day-to-day happenings to future dreams.

Incorporating rituals of connection can also fortify trust and vulnerability. Whether it's a daily gesture like a good-night text or a weekly tradition of sharing a meal without distractions, these acts communicate consistency and appreciation. They signify a shared commitment and attentiveness to each other's emotional worlds.

Ultimately, building trust and vulnerability is an ongoing process. It requires effort, time, and a mutual willingness to be open and honest. But the rewards—a deep, abiding emotional intimacy and a profound connection—are worth every tear, every heartwarming conversation, and every moment of courage. Trust and vulnerability empower partners to truly be seen and loved for who they are, creating a fertile environment for love and desire to thrive.

Emotional Support Techniques

In the realm of emotional intimacy and connection, the ability to offer genuine emotional support can't be understated. It's about creating a safe space where vulnerability thrives and trust blossoms. This involves more than just words; it's the art of being present, both physically and emotionally, and truly empathizing with your partner's experiences. By validating their feelings and offering unwavering support, you build a reservoir of emotional strength that enhances your bond. Encouraging open expression of feelings and fostering empathy isn't just therapeutic; it's transformative. These techniques not only deepen your intimacy but also cultivate a shared emotional resilience, making your partnership a sanctuary of mutual support and love.

Sharing Feelings Openly is a critical pillar under the umbrella of emotional intimacy and connection, serving as a bedrock for fostering genuine closeness between partners. At its core, it's about creating a safe space where both partners feel comfortable expressing their emotions without fear of judgment or backlash. This openness paves the way for a deeper connection and strengthens the emotional bond that often ebbs and flows over time. The act of opening up can be incredibly liberating and healing, allowing couples to navigate their relational landscape with transparency and authenticity.

Imagine shedding the layers of pretense and truly baring your soul to another; that's the kind of openness that builds a strong emotional foundation. It's more than just words—it's about experiencing and validating each other's feelings. Often, emotions can be messy and complicated, but acknowledging them openly can be a profound act of love and acceptance. When partners express vulnerability, it invites empathy, understanding, and ultimately, more profound emotional support. This mutual exchange of genuine sentiments can be transformative, creating a resilient bond that stands the test of time.

In the context of emotional support techniques, sharing feelings openly is not simply about airing grievances or celebrating joys. It's about engaging in meaningful dialogue that promotes mutual respect and compassion. Such interaction requires active listening, empathy, and a willingness to understand where one's partner is coming from. It's crucial to not only share but also to be present and attentive when your partner is doing the same. This approach can enrich your shared experiences and enhance intimacy, turning a relationship into a sanctuary of emotional safety.

Vulnerability, which is a cornerstone of sharing feelings openly, often requires courage and trust. Many find it daunting to articulate their innermost thoughts, fearing rejection or misunderstanding. However, it's important to remember that vulnerability is not a weakness; rather, it's a form of strength that builds deeper connections. By bravely opening up about personal emotional experiences, couples can break down barriers and bridge gaps that might otherwise keep them emotionally distant. This transparency nurtures an understanding that fosters growth, healing, and a more vibrant emotional connection.

Creating an environment that encourages open sharing of feelings involves a blend of patience, empathy, and careful communication. It's about setting the stage for honest conversation and recognising that each partner brings their own emotional experiences and perspectives. Avoiding assumptions and embracing curiosity can play an essential role in this process. By truly listening and responding with compassion, partners can validate each other's emotions, creating a nurturing atmosphere where they can both thrive emotionally.

When feelings are shared openly, it can have a ripple effect on other aspects of the relationship, including libido and physical intimacy. Emotional intimacy and connection are key drivers of desire, as they lay the groundwork for a deeper appreciation and enjoyment of each other's presence. This bond acts as a catalyst for sexual expression, enhancing the overall experience and creating a more fulfilling partnership. Thus, prioritizing emotional openness can be an invaluable technique for rejuvenating the desires and passions within a relationship.

The act of sharing feelings openly also opens pathways for resolution and growth. Conflict is an inevitable part of any relationship, but when partners feel safe to express their emotions, they can address issues with empathy and understanding rather than with defensiveness or hostility. Constructively working through conflicts strengthens the relational fabric and ensures that no resentment lingers beneath the surface. This harmony leads to a more cohesive and durable partnership, allowing love to flourish without the shadows of unresolved issues looming large.

As you embark on the journey of sharing feelings openly with your partner, remember that it's a dynamic process, constantly evolving with time and life changes. Cultivating emotional intimacy takes commitment, effort, and sometimes, learning from past mistakes. Growth in this area can lead to a relationship that not only survives but thrives—serving as a source of joy, comfort, and inspiration. The more willingly you share and embrace each other's emotional worlds, the more rewarding and fulfilling your shared journey becomes.

Empathy in Relationships is the silent thread that weaves itself through the fabric of emotional intimacy, reinforcing the beautiful tapestry of human connection. It's the ability to step into your partner's shoes, to feel their emotions, and to understand their perspectives, which strengthens the bond that keeps a relationship resilient and thriving. In the dance of intimacy, empathy plays a vital role, allowing couples to navigate the complexities of shared life experiences with grace and understanding.

Emotional support is a critical component of any relationship, and empathy serves as its backbone. When a partner feels heard and understood, it creates a nurturing environment where vulnerability is both safe and cherished. Sharing the burden of emotions and offering a shoulder to lean on during challenging times can rejuvenate the soul and renew the connection between partners. The sincerity and warmth conveyed through empathetic interactions can transform everyday encounters into profound exchanges that deepen emotional intimacy.

Practicing empathy isn't limited to moments of crisis or conflict. It's about cultivating a habit of truly seeing and valuing each other in the day-to-day. Whether through actively listening to your partner's day or appreciating their unspoken struggles, small acts of empathy can have a powerful impact. This conscious engagement demonstrates that you don't only hear their words but also feel their unarticulated emotions. In doing so, you affirm their significance and fortify the foundation of your relationship.

Imagine being in a relationship where each partner holds space for the other's emotional experiences, validating feelings and offering compassionate responses. Such a dynamic fosters mutual respect and reinforces trust, pillars essential for emotional intimacy. When partners remain attuned to each other's emotional states and needs, they can preemptively ease tensions and misunderstandings, turning potential conflicts into opportunities for growth and understanding.

Building empathy requires patience, practice, and dedication. It means intentionally slowing down to make room for your partner's emotional reality, sometimes even when it clashes with your own. The journey involves being present, suspending judgment, and offering unconditional support. Practicing this kind of empathetic engagement doesn't just enrich your partner's life; it enriches your own, expanding your emotional range and deepening your connections.

Empathy is also about the willingness to enter difficult emotional territories. It might involve understanding your partner's fears or past traumas, acknowledging their dreams and aspirations, or confronting their insecurities and doubts. This openness to exploring the full spectrum of each other's emotional landscapes creates a partnership that's resilient and adaptive, capable of weathering the storms of life together.

Effective empathy involves both verbal affirmations and nonverbal cues. A gentle touch, a warm embrace, or even a sincere glance can convey profound empathy. These nonverbal elements, coupled with thoughtful words, complete the symphony of emotional understanding that sustains intimacy. It's not just about what you say, but how you say it and how you accompany it with genuine gestures that matter most.

An empathetic relationship fosters an environment where partners are encouraged to grow individually, even as their bond strengthens. It supports both independence and unity, allowing each partner to explore and develop their own needs and desires. When partners feel emotionally supported, they are more inclined to explore and express their own sexual desires, further enhancing the intimate quality of the relationship.

While the journey towards heightened empathy in relationships is ongoing, its rewards are immeasurable. It creates a nurturing emotional landscape where love can flourish uninhibited. As couples practice empathetic engagement, they inevitably foster a love that is robust, adaptable, and enduring. In this shared understanding, partners find not only the essence of emotional intimacy but also the key to a vibrant and fulfilling love life.

Ultimately, empathy transforms relationships from mundane to magical, unveiling layers of meaning and connection that might remain hidden. It invites partners to step outside of themselves and into a shared realm of emotional resonance. Through the practice of empathy, relationships transcend circumstances, blossoming into enduring connections that can brave the evolving nature of life with resilience and grace.

In nurturing empathy, relationships not only survive but thrive, paving the way for true emotional intimacy and connection. The transformative power of empathy lies in its ability to honor the uniqueness and the togetherness of two individuals sharing the journey of life. As you integrate empathy into your emotional support techniques, remember that it's the small, daily choices to listen, understand, and respond with kindness that build a foundation for a deeply satisfying and passionate relationship.

Chapter 6:
Overcoming Common
Barriers to Libido

In the quest for a fuller, more passionate love life, it's crucial to acknowledge and tackle the common hurdles that can dampen desire. Stress and anxiety often loom large, creeping into intimate moments and stifling libido, yet with effective management techniques, these obstacles can be dismantled. Balancing work and personal life is another frequent challenge, where time management and relaxation techniques come into play as vital tools to reclaim time for intimacy and connection. Imagine these barriers as mere shadows lurking in the background—they're disruptors, not permanent fixtures. By embracing practical strategies to navigate life's demands, you're empowering both yourself and your relationship. This journey towards rekindled passion is not just about battling the blockers; it's about celebrating the intimate moments that flourish once those barriers are crossed. Each step forward is a dance towards deeper connection and revitalized desire, underscoring that love is not just a feeling but a practice that thrives with attention and care.

Addressing Stress and Anxiety

In the dance of intimacy, few partners are as unwelcome as stress and anxiety. These two companions can sneak into the bedroom, casting shadows on desire and leaving passion in the cold. Recognizing their presence and addressing them is a vital step in overcoming barriers to a fulfilling libido. Stress and anxiety act as invisible barriers, blocking the path to intimacy and connection. They tighten muscles, distract minds, and distance hearts. To combat these nefarious adversaries, it's essential to understand their origins and arm yourself with strategies to disarm them.

Stress, an inevitable part of modern life, often comes in waves. It can be triggered by work, relationships, finances, or even the pressure to engage intimately. While a little stress is a normal part of life, chronic stress releases a stream of stress hormones such as cortisol, which can wreak havoc on physical and mental health. This physiological response not only dampens desire but also undermines emotional connections with partners. Embracing techniques to manage stress is not just about reducing those harmful hormone levels—it's about reclaiming joy and presence in moments of intimacy.

Anxiety, on the other hand, is the anticipation of future stress and can lead to cycles of worry and fear. Performance anxiety, in particular, can be a significant libido crusher. The fear of not being able to meet a partner's expectations or being compared to past experiences can create an emotional prison. Breaking free requires self-compassion and open communication with your partner. Establishing a foundation of trust where both can express anxieties freely can turn concerns into opportunities for closeness.

To address these barriers, it's crucial to implement mindfulness as a strategy for both stress reduction and anxiety management. Mindfulness encourages you to focus on the present moment, acknowledging feelings without judgment. This practice can be transformative within the context of intimacy. By being fully present, you're not only more in tune with your own needs but also attuned to your partner's, fostering a deeper, more satisfying connection. Simple mindfulness exercises, like deep breathing or guided imagery, can be powerful tools to regain control over intrusive thoughts.

Another potent tool lies in physical activities that enhance both mood and physical health. Exercise has been shown to significantly reduce stress and anxiety levels by releasing endorphins, which act as natural painkillers and mood elevators. Incorporating regular physical activities like yoga or tai chi, which integrate movement with mindful breathing, can do wonders in soothing the nervous system—allowing for a more relaxed and intimate environment.

Adopt a Regular Exercise Routine: Aerobic exercises, strength training, or even a simple daily walk can significantly reduce stress levels. Aligning with your partner's schedule for dual workout sessions could introduce a collective sense of achievement and partnership.

Engage in Relaxation Practices: Practices like deep breathing, progressive muscle relaxation, or guided meditation can be an oasis of calm amid a bustling day. Sharing a meditation session with your partner might also introduce a novel, calming component to your routine.

Create Rituals for Unwinding: Establish shared rituals for increasing relaxation and reducing stress, like having a cup of herbal tea together in the evening, which can also reinforce your bond.

The act of unwinding should not be underestimated. Creating a tranquil bedtime ritual or turning the bedroom into a stress-free zone can signal to your mind and body that it's time to relax and connect. Evoking a sense of ritual can delineate daily stressors from an intimate environment, making the transition from daily life to romantic interlude seamless.

It's also essential to carve out moments for genuine communication with your partner. Discussing both shared and individual stressors openly can diffuse tension and foster mutual support. Even brief check-ins can reinforce that you're a team, capable of tackling life's hurdles together. This kind of emotional collaboration not only strengthens the relationship but also diminishes stress's grip on your shared intimate experiences.

However, when stress and anxiety become overwhelming, seeking professional guidance can provide a structured path to healing. A therapist can offer both partners techniques and interventions tailored to their specific needs, helping them develop tools to manage stress and anxiety more effectively. Sometimes, simply having an objective voice can illuminate new pathways for building a resilient, joyful connection.

Ultimately, while stress and anxiety can loom large, they're not insurmountable. By addressing them with intention and compassion, it's possible to clear the path to desire, rediscover connection, and foster an environment where passion thrives unencumbered. In doing so, couples can transform potential obstacles into opportunities for growth, intimacy, and renewed vitality in their shared journey.

Managing Work-Life Balance

In the relentless whirl of modern life, managing work-life balance becomes a pivotal act of self-love that holds the power to rejuvenate your libido and deepen intimacy with your partner. It's about crafting a life where work commitments and personal passions don't just coexist but complement each other. By navigating the delicate dance between career pressures and personal fulfillment, you can carve out space for romance and desire. Prioritizing time management and embracing relaxation techniques not only reduce stress but also free up mental and emotional bandwidth, making space for intimacy to thrive. In fostering a harmonious balance, you redefine success not just by professional achievements but also by the strength and satisfaction of your intimate connections. This intricate balancing act can reignite the spark that adds a profound layer of joy and contentment to your shared journey.

Time Management Tips can be a lifeline when the intricate dance of managing work-life balance threatens to overshadow the deeper connections we crave. Juggling professional responsibilities and personal relationships often feels like a high-wire act, where one misstep might cause a tumble into neglected desires and strained intimacy. Addressing this balancing act is not just about blocking off hours; it's about cultivating a mindset that prioritizes love as much as labor.

Start by redefining what "balance" means to you and your partner. It's easy to get trapped in the idea that perfect symmetry between work and personal life exists, but perhaps it's more about ebb and flow. Some days, work will demand more, and on others, personal time will take the spotlight. The key is flexibility—being okay with occasional imbalance and knowing when to shift focus. This mindset not only eases pressure but also enhances connection by fostering communication about shifting needs.

Set boundaries both at work and home. It's all too tempting to let the workday extend into personal time, thinking you'll just "finish this one last thing." However, unchecked, this becomes a habit that eats away at quality time with your partner. Create clear cutoffs for when work ends and home life begins. Communicate these boundaries to colleagues if necessary, ensuring they respect your personal time as much as you do.

Utilize scheduling as a tool to safeguard relationship time. Often, we think intimacy should be spontaneous, but with busy lives, scheduled intimacy can be equally rewarding. Set aside regular intervals dedicated to each other. Be it a weekly date night or a simple coffee chat at home, these moments create expectation and excitement. They become anchors amidst the chaos, reminding you both that despite demanding weeks, you are prioritizing each other's company.

Consider the use of micro-moments, tiny pockets of time that can morph into meaningful interaction. Not everything requires significant hours blocked on a calendar. Send a loving text during a break or share a joke over lunch. These snippets of intimacy are manageable in any schedule and can fortify the bond without waiting for larger, planned segments of time. It's about presence, not duration.

Technology can either be a burden or a boon in this quest for balance; harness it wisely. Use calendars and reminders to keep personal commitments top of mind, just as you would for work obligations. Consider apps that encourage mindfulness or couples' apps that facilitate intimate conversations even when apart. Yet, be mindful to disconnect when it's time to connect in person—put the devices away and give undivided attention to each other.

Beyond tangible steps, underlying all these actions is a commitment to see personal and relationship time as investments, not indulgences. Whether it's a hobby shared together, a lazy Sunday morning embraced fully, or even undisturbed quiet time side by side, these are the spaces where desire can flourish naturally. They're not just breaks from the grind; they're the essential touchstones of a shared life.

Finally, recognize the necessity of self-care within this balance. When you're well, you bring a healthier, more centered self to your partner and to your shared moments. Encourage one another to have personal downtime to recharge, which in turn enriches the quality of the time spent together. Being truly balanced often means taking turns supporting each other's times of fulfillment, creating a symphony where both parts thrive in harmony.

Embrace these time management tips not merely as techniques but as a journey towards intentionally entwining love and life. In nurturing this delicate dance, the path open to rekindle desire and deepen intimacy within a partnership becomes not only possible but beautifully rewarding.

Relaxation Techniques as they pertain to managing work-life balance, can be an essential tool in overcoming common barriers to libido, particularly when the pressures of modern life weigh heavily on intimacy and desire. In a world that often demands more than it gives back, finding moments of calm and tranquility can feel like a distant dream. Yet, relaxation isn't just a serene escape; it's a vital way to rejuvenate your senses, enabling a harmonious balance between work obligations and personal fulfillment.

The first step towards integrating relaxation into your daily routine is acknowledging its importance. Stress is a pervasive force that can sap your energy and diminish your enthusiasm for intimacy. By regularly practicing relaxation techniques, you not only reduce stress but also create a welcoming space for desire to flourish. When you're relaxed, your body produces happier hormones, which naturally boost your libido. An essential technique is deep breathing. This simple, yet powerful method involves inhaling deeply, holding for a moment, and then exhaling slowly. By focusing on your breath, you can calm your mind, ease worry, and refocus your energy—a foundation that strengthens your intimate connections.

Visualization is another potent technique for cultivating relaxation. Imagine a scene that embodies tranquility, whether it's a serene beach at sunset or a quiet forest after a rainfall. Close your eyes and immerse yourself in that environment, letting the peace wash over you. By engaging all your senses, visualization not only pulls you away from workplace demands but also invites an inner calm that enhances your connection with your partner. Moreover, sharing this visualization exercise with your partner can heighten your shared experience and deepen your bond.

The art of progressive muscle relaxation is an often overlooked, yet effective relaxation technique. It involves systematically tensing and relaxing different muscle groups, beginning from your head and moving down to your toes. This practice enhances body awareness and alleviates the tension that often accompanies hectic work schedules. As you release the physical stress, mental calm follows, creating a fertile ground where intimacy and desire can reside peacefully. Practicing this technique as part of your evening routine can transition your mind from work mode to a more nurturing, intimate state.

Incorporating yoga and meditation into your weekly routine can be transformative. The physical flow of yoga helps release pent-up tension in your muscles, promotes better posture, and improves circulation—all crucial for a healthy libido. Meanwhile, meditation sharpens your focus, allowing you to remain present and responsive to your partner's needs. Both practices facilitate a deeper connection with your body, enabling you to tune into its signals and respond with clarity and compassion, which are essential for cultivating passion and desire.

Mindfulness is a key factor in relaxation, urging you to live in the moment rather than fretting over past mishaps or future duties. Embrace mindfulness by engaging fully in whatever you're doing, whether it's savoring a meal, appreciating a piece of music, or simply enjoying a quiet moment with your partner. By grounding yourself in the present, you'll find that the daily grind fades away, leaving room for an intimate connection to blossom.

Introducing aromatherapy into your home can further enrich your relaxation experience. Scents such as lavender, chamomile, and sandalwood are known for their calming effects. Whether diffused in a room or used as a part of a relaxing massage, these scents can transform your space into a haven of tranquility, soothing frazzled nerves and setting a scene ripe for romance.

Scheduling and commitment are vital components of successfully implementing relaxation techniques to balance work and personal life. Just as you would schedule a business meeting, allocate specific times in your week dedicated solely to relaxation. Whether it's an hour-long yoga class or a 20-minute evening meditation, treating these sessions as non-negotiable can create a rhythm that supports both your professional obligations and your personal well-being.

Finally, remember the power of nature in achieving relaxation. Spending time outdoors, even if it's just a short walk in a park, can significantly reduce stress and anxiety. Nature's beauty and tranquility provide a much-needed refuge from the electronics and pressures of everyday life, fostering a mental reset that invigorates both your body and spirit. Fresh air and natural surroundings facilitate openness and warmth, easing the path to intimacy.

Incorporating relaxation techniques into your lifestyle isn't just about managing stress; it's about enriching your life with moments of peace and connection. When work-life balance feels right, and tension is managed, your libido is more likely to thrive. Allow these techniques to guide you toward a more intimate, fulfilling relationship, not just with your partner, but with yourself as well. By prioritizing relaxation, you're investing in the happiness and health of your relationship—a choice that ultimately paves the way for lasting passion and joy.

Chapter 7:
The Power of Touch and Sensuality

Touch is an unspoken language that can ignite passion and deepen intimacy, making it a powerful tool in any relationship. It transcends words, offering an exquisite dance of connection through the tender mapping of each other's bodies. Sensuality starts with the fingertips, tracing invisible paths that venture into worlds of pleasure yet undiscovered. Every touch carries potential, opening gateways to feelings of comfort, trust, and excitement. When you embark on the journey to explore each other's erogenous zones, you invite a new form of communication, one that beckons closeness and vulnerability. This exploration requires patience and attentiveness, transforming simple caresses into profound experiences that speak directly to the heart and soul. The warmth of skin against skin and the delicate art of massage create a sanctuary where both partners can unite, explore, and celebrate their shared physical and emotional landscapes, fostering a bond that reaches beyond the ordinary.

The Art of Sensual Massage

Executing the art of sensual massage isn't just about learning technique—it's about creating an environment where two people can feel comfortable, loved, and open to connection. The real power of sensual massage lies not only in the physical touch but also in the emotional and psychological closeness it fosters. A massage can become a profound act of love, a dance of hands over skin that defies words. It's an unspoken conversation between partners—a tactile language that expresses care, attention, and desire. This is more than mere routine; it's a pathway to rediscovering intimacy.

To set the scene, consider the ambiance. Lower the lights, perhaps illuminate the room with candles for a soft glow. Choose music that resonates with both of you, rhythms that entwine with your heartbeats. Warm the room to a comfortable temperature to allow undistracted immersion into the experience. The fragrances chosen should be pleasing to both, maybe a hint of lavender or jasmine, elevating the senses without overwhelming them. Atmosphere can be as powerful as touch itself in creating an inviting space.

Now, consider the tactile exploration. Use oils that suit your partner's skin, maybe something silkily luxuriant that glides smoothly. The choice of oil can enhance the sensory delight, providing both glide and nourishment to the skin. The scent of the oil should complement the room's aromas—subtle enough to linger in memory but not dominate the air.

Begin with a simple touch, laying your hands gently on your partner's back or shoulders without applying pressure, allowing your skin to absorb warmth and energy. This first step is about presence, about signaling that this moment is dedicated to your shared connection. From there, let your hands wander, exploring with soft strokes, gentle kneads, and loving caresses. The pressure should be varied according to your partner's preferences—light to invigorate, deep to relax.

A remarkable aspect of sensual massage is how it encourages partners to communicate wordlessly. As your hands move, listen to their body's responses: a soft moan, a sigh of contentment, or a shift in position. Silence can be profound; it's a space where bodies speak a language of their own, free from misunderstandings that words sometimes bring. Encourage feedback but let the silence speak too. It's a time for exploration and adaptation, letting touch guide you.

We mustn't neglect the less obvious parts of the body that can add a uniquely personal dimension to this experience. Explore areas often ignored in daily life—scalp, elbows, calves. Each inch of the body tells a story of tension, pleasure, or overlooked sensitivity. Tailoring your touch to these often missed areas can bring added pleasure and connection, as your partner realizes how fully and deeply observed they are.

Sensual massage embraces the art of slowness. In a world in constant motion, this is a space for stillness, for ensuring that the act itself is an embrace of the present moment. As life rushes by, this moment is a celebration of being together, here and now. Slowing the pace of your hands can slow the world, creating an almost meditative state where both partners can find greater connection to each other.

The mind isn't absent in this tactile journey. Both process and result, massaging your partner is also about how both of you feel throughout. Power lies not just in the physical act but in the psychological relaxation it brings. Feelings of safety, trust, and vulnerability can nurture the kind of bond that's so much more than skin deep.

Incorporate variation with creative touches—maybe the soft caress of a feather or the gentle stroke with fingertips. Understanding how different textures can spark or deepen the experience, you begin to build a repertoire of gestures, each imbued with personal meaning. It becomes a dance of spontaneity and craft, a fluid movement that evolves as you continue to explore each other's preferences and desires.

Feel free to experiment too with the pace and rhythm of your caresses, ebbing and flowing with the conversation of your bodies. You may incorporate inspirations from other styles, like the invigorating strokes of Swedish massage, the focused attention of trigger point, or the deeply enveloping movements of an Esalen style. Merging these into your own personal narrative of touch reflects the deep connection you share with your partner.

Above all, remember this isn't about mastering a skill; it's about opening a space to feel, to explore, to laugh, and even to stumble at times in the pursuit of closeness. The art of sensual massage transforms the mundane into the extraordinary, embedding its practitioners in a timeless exchange of warmth and affection.

This practice, honed in love and attention, isn't just a technique— it's an ongoing dialogue that can radically transform the connection between couples. Sensual massage can soften everyday stress, tear down the barriers of routine, and remind us of touch's healing power. More than just a prelude to more intimate engagement, it is a fulfilling closeness that stands beautifully on its own.

Ultimately, the art of sensual massage lies not only in the touch itself but in the embrace of one another—in mind, body, and heart. It connects desire with intention, fostering a deep-seated bond that enhances every facet of intimacy, breathing life into every shared moment. This is the pathway we all seek, a most potent reminder of the sanctity and power of human connection through touch.

Exploring Erogenous Zones

In the journey to deepen intimacy and enhance desire, exploring erogenous zones offers a thrilling adventure into the power of touch. These sensory-rich areas of the body, when kissed or caressed, can ignite passion and heighten pleasure in ways that words alone often can't convey. From the nape of the neck to the soles of the feet, discovering each other's erogenous zones is not just about physical contact—it's about emotional connection and mutual exploration. As you navigate these intimate territories, pay close attention to your partner's responses, allowing their reactions to guide you toward what feels most pleasurable and connective. Don't be afraid to communicate openly, such as whispering desires and feedback, which turns the experience into a shared dialogue of affection and vulnerability. By tuning into these cues and savoring the journey, partners can weave a tapestry of erotic energy that not only tantalizes the senses but also strengthens the bonds of love and intimacy.

Identifying Erogenous Zones represents an intimate exploration of the body's incredible ability to experience pleasure, offering a deeper connection between partners. These zones serve as gateways to heightened arousal and emotional bonding, allowing individuals to engage in a dance of touch and sensation that fuels desire. Understanding the unique landscape of erogenous zones is essential, as each person's body is a distinctive map, ready to be discovered and celebrated.

We often think of certain areas—the lips, neck, and inner thighs—as universal erogenous zones, and indeed they play significant roles. However, each individual possesses a personalized array of hotspots that might surprise both them and their partner. The key to unlocking these zones lies in curiosity and a willingness to explore and communicate openly. This journey is less about conforming to general knowledge and more about unlocking what makes each person feel desired and cherished.

Our skin houses millions of nerve endings, with some regions wired more densely than others. The heightened sensitivity of these zones means that even the lightest touch can evoke strong reactions. Starting with the commonly known areas can be an excellent way to build initial confidence. Testing out gentle kisses, soft caresses, or even a light blow of air can reveal which areas elicit the strongest responses. Partners who engage in this discovery process cultivate a deeper trust and intimacy, knowing that they're sharing something profoundly personal.

When trying to identify these zones, one effective method is to incorporate touch into everyday interactions, allowing reactions to guide the journey. This relaxed, unscheduled exploration can maintain a sense of spontaneity that often enhances excitement. Keeping the atmosphere playful and pressure-free is crucial, as stress and expectation can dampen the experience. A playful whisper, an adventurous spirit, and a touch of humor can go a long way in making the process enjoyable for both partners.

While the physical aspect of identifying erogenous zones is deeply important, mental and emotional receptiveness should not be overlooked. An individual's psychological state can greatly influence their physical responsiveness. Emotional safety, open communication, and mutual respect lay the groundwork for successful exploration. Discussing boundaries, desires, and preferences before and during this process ensures that both partners feel valued and understood, promoting both mutual respect and consent.

Of course, the art of exploring erogenous zones extends beyond simple touch. Including other senses can amplify the experience. Consider incorporating aromatic oils or scented candles to engage the sense of smell. Soft, sensual music can enhance the auditory experience, setting the mood and helping both partners relax into the moment. Coordinating these elements helps create a multi-sensory environment that enriches the journey.

The journey of discovery can also benefit from a touch of the exotic and the unknown. Incorporate tools or toys designed to stimulate specific areas—a feather, silk scarf, or even temperature play with ice cubes or warm oils can introduce novel sensations to areas already identified as erogenous zones. This can lead to even richer experiences and nuance in connection.

Understanding that these zones can shift and change over time adds another layer to the experience. What might be intensely pleasurable at one stage of life could evolve or fade, only to be reignited in new ways later on. Maintaining a lifelong curiosity and willingness to explore with your partner keeps the spark alive and ensures your intimate connection continues to grow and transform with time.

Ultimately, identifying erogenous zones is about more than just pinpointing parts of the body that feel good when touched. It's a collaborative adventure of discovery that can deepen emotional bonds and elevate the overall experience of intimacy in a relationship. Approach it with openness, creativity, and a generous spirit, and the rewards will be shared moments of exceptional joy and connection.

How to Utilize Erogenous Zones lies at the heart of deepening connections through physical touch and sensuality. This facet of intimacy involves more than just discovering sensitive areas; it opens a world where physical interactions transcend into deeply emotional connections. Understanding and responding to erogenous zones can transform not just your love life but also the mutual understanding between partners, fostering a richer, more fulfilling intimacy.

Engaging with erogenous zones is akin to playing a beautiful melody on a finely tuned instrument, where each note resonates with your partner's unique rhythm. Start by tuning into subtle signals and reactions, allowing your touch to communicate the tenderness and curiosity you hold for one another. It's about patience and attention, allowing desire to rise with each gentle caress, turning anticipation into a shared experience.

To fully harness the power of these sensitive areas, it's important to approach each encounter with a sense of adventure and wonder, treating it as uncharted territory ripe for exploration. Some zones might be universally recognized, while others are uniquely personal, varying greatly between individuals. This combination of general knowledge and personalized discovery allows partners to decide what feels right and invigorating.

Encouraging your partner to express what feels good strengthens your bond and expands your intimate vocabulary. It's like learning a new language where each word, each phrase communicates affection and understanding. Approach each exploration with open-hearted curiosity, and don't shy away from asking gentle questions or offering comforting affirmations to guide your actions and reactions to better tailor your touch.

Sometimes, recognizing erogenous zones can begin with the delicate areas commonly cherished—the nape of the neck, inner thighs, or along the spine, where science reveals high concentrations of nerve endings. However, the true art lies in turning the known into new sensations by varying the pressure, speed, and temperature of your touch while paying special attention to your partner's cues.

You might find that adding a sense of surprise can elevate the sensation beyond the physical. Perhaps a trailing kiss or a light touch becomes exhilarating when unexpected, leading to heightened anticipation and connection. The thrill of what's coming next can become just as pleasurable as the touch itself, building a narrative of intimacy rooted deeply in your shared experiences.

Utilizing different textures can also add depth to the experience. Introduce silk, feathers, or even ice cubes to awaken the senses. These sensory elements can create unique experiences, opening new pathways of excitement and anticipation. Invitations to explore with closed eyes can further heighten sensitivity, making each touch more pronounced and meaningful.

Remember, exploration is a two-way street that can lead to surprising revelations about each other. Approach this journey as partners crafting a story—a story filled with playful exploration and reassuring touches that speak volumes about desire and care. Learning how erogenous zones respond to different stimuli can bolster trust, as it requires an openness and willingness to understand your partner's pleasures deeply

It is vital to recognize that these explorations shouldn't be rushed. Letting moments linger ensures neither partner feels pressured, and instead, both become enveloped in the tenderness of being present with each other. The essence of the act is being together, sharing each moment's warmth and delight—whether it leads to playful laughter or silent awe.

Finally, it's crucial to honor boundaries and ensure both partners feel comfortable at all times. Communication is paramount, both verbally and through non-verbal cues, asking for consent and check-ins along the way. This ensures that the journey remains enjoyable and consensual, creating a safe space for both partners to freely express themselves.

In conclusion, learning how to utilize erogenous zones is a journey of discovery and creativity between partners. It's about understanding each other's bodies and minds in the quest for deeper connection and pleasure. By embracing this journey with an open heart and mind, you nurture a relationship filled with warmth, empathy, and boundless love.

Chapter 8:
Sexual Techniques and Practices

Chapter 8 delves into the exciting realm of sexual techniques and practices, unveiling how to elevate your intimate experiences to new heights. Through the exploration of new positions and techniques, this chapter inspires partners to embrace the art of experimentation, enhancing pleasure and deepening their connection. Foreplay is underscored not just as a precursor but as an essential component of passionate encounters, where the emphasis is on mindful and mutual engagement. Encouraging creativity and an open mind, the chapter guides couples to discover what brings them joy, fostering an environment where both partners feel heard and fulfilled. Amidst the journey of shared exploration, the importance of communication and consent remains paramount, as these are the keys to forging an intimate bond that thrives on trust and mutual pleasure. Ultimately, this chapter is a celebration of sexual curiosity and togetherness, motivating lovers to continually find new ways to delight each other in a dance as unique as their connection.

New Positions and Techniques

In the realm of intimacy, novelty can serve as a powerful catalyst for reigniting passion and deepening connection. Exploring new positions and techniques is much like venturing into uncharted territories together, discovering what feels right and what elevates pleasure. This exploration isn't just about trying every position known to humankind but about finding what uniquely resonates with you and your partner, enhancing your shared moments with creativity and affection.

One approach to breathe new life into your intimate moments is to revisit what might have become routine. Consider this: slight adjustments in angle, pace, or environment can transform a familiar experience into something fresh and invigorating. Sometimes, a gentle tweak to a classic favorite position can unlock new sensations. One partner might find deeper pleasure from shifting leg placement or changing the rhythm of movement. It's this spirit of curiosity and willingness that underpins the journey of discovery together.

Engaging in such explorations requires a foundation of trust and clear communication. It's about ensuring that both partners feel comfortable expressing their boundaries and desires. This open dialogue lays the groundwork for exploring unconventional positions that can break free from routine patterns. Introducing elements such as props or supports can aid in achieving different poses and can be particularly helpful when trying positions that require greater flexibility or strength.

Think of props like strategically positioned pillows, which can elevate certain body parts to achieve deeper angles or support tired muscles. Remember, props aren't about complicating the act; they're there to enhance comfort and creativity. Kneeling positions like the renowned but often underexplored "Lotus" can be invigorated by a sensual backdrop, perhaps with soft lighting or comforting scents, creating an immersive atmosphere that envelops the senses.

Take your exploration further by considering positions that encourage face-to-face connection, such as sitting positions where partners straddle each other. These intimate arrangements foster a sense of closeness and eye contact, amplifying the emotional connection and allowing for meaningful expressions beyond words.

It's in these shared gazes and undistracted focus on one another that profound bonds are often cultivated.

The journey through new positions isn't strictly about physicality; it's about the emotional and mental energy you bring into the encounter. The spontaneity of trying something new can rekindle excitement, while the shared laughter over an attempted yet comical placement can reinforce companionship. It's vital to retain a sense of humor and not take the exploration too seriously, remembering it's about mutual enjoyment, not achieving perfection.

Furthermore, consider integrating gentle movements such as rocking or subtle sliding motions within a position, which can introduce a rhythmic dance to the interaction. The "Coital Alignment Technique" (CAT), for instance, builds on modifying the traditional missionary position by focusing on a rocking motion that enhances clitoral stimulation and synchronous pleasure, showing how a nuanced perspective on positioning can lead to rewarding outcomes.

Staying grounded in the practice requires patience and a willingness to adapt. Bodies are dynamic, and what works one day might need adjustment the next. It's about tuning into each other's signals and being responsive to them. Encourage a language of affirmative feedback—simple phrases like "That feels good," or "Can we try this?" can constructively guide each other through the intimate dance.

In addition to expanding your repertoire of positions, embracing the art of sensual teasing can elevate anticipation and pleasure. Consider prolonging foreplay with tantalizing touch or exploring techniques such as temperature play, where contrasting sensations can heighten awareness and heighten senses. This initial build-up, often ripe with expectancy, can transform the actual act into an explosive crescendo of shared delight.

Remember, at the heart of exploring new positions and techniques is the pursuit of shared pleasure, not just individual satisfaction. It's this mutual willingness to journey together, to explore without fear and embrace the vulnerabilities that arise, that can lead to richer experiences. Ultimately, it's about celebrating the unique sensual language you and your partner have cultivated, savored through creativity and love.

In conclusion, every new position or technique adopted should be filtered through a lens of mutual respect and consensual experimentation. There are no definitive rules except what you and your partner agree upon. Dive into these explorations with a sense of adventure, recognizing that the encounters hold the potential to weave new threads into the fabric of your relationship, strengthening the tapestry of intimacy and affection you share.

Enhancing Pleasure for Both Partners

Unlocking deeper pleasure for both partners in a relationship isn't just about mastering new techniques, but rather embracing a mindful and empathetic approach to shared intimacy. The key lies in being attentive to each other's body language and responses, which can reveal much about desires and comfort levels. Consider integrating playful exploration and open-minded experimentation, as this invites not just physical satisfaction but emotional bonding, too. A journey toward sensual fulfillment is a dance of mutual appreciation and giving, where both partners feel safe and empowered to express their needs. By fostering an environment where curiosity and trust thrive, couples can create rich, shared experiences that deepen connection and heighten the joy of being together. The emphasis should always be on discovery and pleasure, not on achieving a specific outcome, as the former nurtures continual growth and harmony in your partnership.

Techniques for Foreplay are a vital part of any intimate relationship, creating a foundation for deeper connection and heightened pleasure between partners. Foreplay isn't just about preparing for what comes next; it's an art form in its own right, designed to cultivate desire and deepen emotional bonds. By encouraging both partners to engage fully in the present moment, it allows for a more connected and fulfilling experience. When done thoughtfully, foreplay can transform the sexual experience from a simple act into an intimate exchange where both partners feel valued and cherished.

To truly enhance pleasure for both partners, foreplay should be seen as a dance, where rhythm and variation keep the experience lively and engaging. Start by focusing on the senses, awakening each with an array of gentle yet tantalizing touches. It's essential to recognize that foreplay is not a one-size-fits-all activity but one that should be customized to fit the unique tastes and desires of both individuals involved. Slowly embracing and discovering each other's bodies can build anticipation and excitement, setting the stage for more intense experiences.

Effective communication is foundational in foreplay. This doesn't only mean verbal communication, although talking about preferences, desires, and boundaries can indeed heighten the experience. Non-verbal cues are just as important; learning to read your partner's body language and responding to subtle signals can help you understand what they truly crave. The anticipation built during this time can be as thrilling as the actual act, making it important to explore these moments patiently and with focused attention.

Variety in technique is crucial in keeping foreplay stimulating. Try experimenting with different types of touch, varying from gentle caresses to more deliberate pressure, depending on what seems to elicit the most response. Introducing elements like feathers, silk scarves, or even simple variations in temperature can engage the senses in novel ways and introduce an adventurous aspect to your sensual repertoire. It's essential to keep an open mind and be willing to try new methods, continuously exploring what keeps your partner intrigued.

Oral stimulation often plays a pivotal role in foreplay, and it can be tailored to enhance pleasure distinctively. By focusing on erogenous zones and alternating between fast and slow, light and firm touches, couples can discover new levels of enjoyment. It's vital to stay attuned to your partner's feedback, both verbal and non-verbal, and to explore together—not every technique will work for every person, but finding what ignites your partner's desire can lead to extraordinary moments of intimacy.

Incorporating massage into your foreplay routine can also offer immense benefits, not only as a means of relaxation but also as a method to deepen your connection. The act of massaging can be incredibly intimate, allowing both partners to explore each other's bodies in a nurturing and caring manner. Warm oils or lotions can add a sensory element that further enhances the experience, providing an avenue for mutual relaxation and the release of pent-up tension.

Vocal expressions can also be a powerful part of foreplay, even if just through subtle moans or affirmations of enjoyment. By openly expressing pleasure and excitement, couples can create an environment of mutual encouragement, where each partner feels free to explore their desires. Engaging in a dialogue about what feels good in the moment can clarify intentions and ensure satisfaction for both parties, nurturing a stronger, more unified intimate bond.

Remember, the mind itself is also a potent tool for foreplay. Setting the scene for seduction begins in the mind. Whether through flirtatious texts exchanged throughout the day or setting up a romantic environment with candles and mood-setting music, anticipation can build powerfully long before any physical touch occurs. This psychological build-up is integral to heightening the eventual physical encounter and ensures a more passionate expression of love.

Foreplay's ultimate goal is to enhance the overall experience of intimacy. It should never be rushed or overlooked, as it lays the groundwork for mutual fulfillment and heightened connection. Through a blend of communication, exploration, and attentive presence, each partner can feel more attuned to the other's psyche and body, making each encounter a step closer to achieving deeper levels of satisfaction and connection.

In conclusion, the art of foreplay is an essential element in the tapestry of a healthy and vibrant sexual relationship. It is a practice where creativity, patience, and attentiveness converge, fostering an environment where both partners can explore and rejuvenate their mutual desire. As you invest in these practices, may you find that foreplay becomes not just an initiation to intimacy, but a deeply enriching and enjoyable journey all its own.

Importance of Experimentation In the realm of sexuality, experimentation isn't just a playful suggestion; it's a fundamental aspect of enhancing the shared pleasure between partners. Embracing experimentation invites a world of possibilities that can deepen both intimacy and satisfaction. So why is experimentation so crucial in this sacred dance of connection? Simply put, it's about discovery—finding what makes each other tick, embracing new experiences, and keeping the sparks flying. By venturing into the unknown together, couples can break free from routine and reignite their passion, leading to a more fulfilling relationship.

Variety is the spice of life, as they say, and when it comes to sexual techniques, that variety can lead to richer and more satisfying experiences. Experimentation can be as simple as trying new positions or as adventurous as exploring different environments. The idea is not just about physical variation but about mental engagement as well.

Engaging in new practices can stimulate the senses in unexpected ways and foster a deeper emotional connection. The anticipation that comes with trying something new generates excitement, enhancing the overall experience for both partners.

Experimentation also creates a fertile ground for communication. When couples explore new techniques and practices, they open the door to honest conversations about likes and dislikes. In doing so, they strengthen their communication skills and build trust. Partners who are willing to share their fantasies and preferences are more likely to feel understood and cared for, which is foundational to a thriving sexual partnership. Discussing what works or what doesn't in a supportive and nonjudgmental way helps both individuals feel safer to express themselves more fully.

Adventure in the bedroom can tackle the monotony that sometimes seeps into a long-term relationship. Trying something different disrupts the usual patterns and invigorates the senses, refocusing partners on one another in new, exhilarating ways. Even minor changes—like lighting, music, or even role-play—might be enough to turn predictability on its head and make intimacy fresh again. Experimentation in sexual practices calls for both courage and vulnerability, and through this, partners can cultivate a shared sense of curiosity and openness.

Moreover, experimentation can play a key role in solving issues of mismatched libidos. It allows couples to explore new forms of foreplay and find activities that might be more stimulating for one partner, thus bridging the desire gap. For many, certain techniques or scenarios can be more arousing, and these preferences can be uncovered through experimentation. This creative exploration turns what could be a stumbling block in intimacy into an opportunity for growth and understanding.

The role of experimentation as a path to enhancing pleasure also extends to discovering erogenous zones that may have previously gone unnoticed. The human body is a treasure trove of sensations waiting to be explored, and a spirit of experimentation makes this discovery process an exciting journey. As partners explore these hidden regions together, they can create an atmospheres of wonder and exploration, vastly enriching their sexual experiences.

It's essential to remember that experimentation does not always mean trying extreme things. It's about incremental changes and the willingness to see where those changes might lead. It's also about allowing space for laughter and mistakes, understanding that not every new experience will hit the mark. The beauty of it lies in the process— the shared adventure, the learning, and the communication that come with trying something new together.

Safety and mutual consent, however, are paramount. As couples embark on their exploratory adventures, establishing boundaries and ensuring comfortable communication is critical. Both partners should feel valued and heard, able to voice their level of comfort with particular activities without fear of judgment or dismissal. This mutual respect fosters an environment where experimentation is not only pleasurable but also secure and nurturing.

When partners feel safe and secure, they're more likely to open themselves up to new experiences and ways of connecting. The importance of experimentation in enhancing pleasure lies not just in the acts themselves but in the emotional intimacy they can cultivate. It's about growing together, discovering new layers of each other's desires, and building a more resilient bond.

In conclusion, the importance of experimentation in sexual techniques and practices cannot be overstated when it comes to enhancing pleasure for both partners. The willingness to innovate and explore nourishes the emotional and physical paths of intimacy, ensuring a dynamic and deeply satisfying connection. As each new experiment unfolds, couples reveal layers of passion and curiosity, writing their unique love stories, chapter by adventurous chapter.

Chapter 9:
Reigniting Passion in Long-Term Relationships

In the dynamic tapestry of long-term relationships, reigniting passion can feel like a grand, heartfelt dance that continuously evolves. For couples who've been together for a considerable time, the spark can feel dimmed by routine and familiarity, but this doesn't mean the fire is extinguished. It calls for a conscious weaving of romantic gestures and spontaneous surprises into the everyday, allowing desire to flourish anew. Picture planning a date night that whisks you both away from the mundane, perhaps to a cherished spot or a delightful new adventure that stirs excitement. Small, unexpected acts of love—a handwritten note, a favorite dish prepared without notice, or an unexpected embrace—can infuse fresh energy into the bond you share. By placing value on keeping the spark alive, you nurture not just passion, but a deeper, more intimate connection that binds two souls intricately and eternally, rekindling the warmth that first brought you together.

Keeping the Spark Alive

Long-term relationships are beautiful in their depth and complexity, but keeping the spark alive often requires intentional action and mindful nurturing. While the shared history between partners can be a strong foundation, familiarity sometimes leads to complacency. In such relationships, maintaining excitement and passion can be as challenging as it is rewarding. This section will explore practical strategies for reigniting passion, offering techniques and insights designed to keep the flame burning in long-term partnerships.

Variety is key when it comes to infusing excitement into a partnership. Trying new activities together can stimulate the brain and foster a sense of adventure that reignites desire. Engaging in novel experiences helps break the monotony, reminding partners of the joy that initially drew them to each other. Whether it's a cooking class, a dance lesson, or an out-of-town adventure, new experiences can create fresh memories and deepen the bond.

Small acts of love can also have a significant impact on maintaining passion. Romantic gestures don't need to be grandiose to be effective. A heartfelt note left on the car dashboard or a surprise breakfast in bed can communicate affection and appreciation. These gestures serve as daily reminders of the cherished feelings that might sometimes get lost in everyday life. The element of surprise can add an unexpected depth to ordinary moments, turning the mundane into magical.

Dedicated time for one another is vital in keeping a relationship vibrant. Planning regular date nights, for example, ensures that the couple steps away from the whirlwind of responsibilities and focuses solely on each other. These moments foster intimacy and can be as simple or extravagant as desired. What matters most is the intent behind them—a commitment to prioritizing the relationship amidst the hustle and bustle of life.

Communication remains a fundamental component of sustaining passion. Open dialogues about desires and emotional needs can nurture a deeper understanding between partners. This involves not only speaking but also actively listening to each other. Practicing empathy in these conversations builds emotional closeness, creating a safe space where both individuals feel valued and understood.

Incorporating touch into daily interactions can significantly enhance connection. Touch is a powerful form of non-verbal communication that can convey warmth, comfort, and desire. Simple acts like holding hands, a gentle back rub, or a tender kiss can reignite the physical connection that is sometimes overshadowed by routine. Physical intimacy helps maintain a strong bond, reinforcing emotional ties through the language of touch.

Set aside moments for reflection and appreciation. Amidst the busyness of life, it can be easy to take partners for granted. By consciously acknowledging and expressing gratitude for one another, couples can strengthen their bond. This practice not only highlights the positives within the relationship but also encourages continued effort from both parties to nurture the spark.

Challenges and changes are inevitable in any relationship. Circumstances such as career shifts, relocations, or personal growth can impact the dynamic between partners. Approaching these changes with a flexible mindset can help maintain passion. Viewing challenges as opportunities for growth and adaptation reinforces resilience in the relationship. Embracing change together can even deepen the connection as partners navigate through life's ups and downs collaboratively.

Rekindling passion in a long-term relationship is akin to tending a garden. It requires careful attention, intentional care, and a willingness to continually grow and adapt. By embracing creativity, communication, and connection, couples can transform their relationships into lifelong adventures filled with love and desire. Maintaining the spark is not about holding onto the past but about continuously aspiring to new ways of loving each other.

Ultimately, the key to keeping the spark alive lies in never losing sight of the reasons that brought the couple together. Cherishing the journey, along with its shared experiences and challenges, cultivates a landscape of love that can reignite passion even in the longest partnerships. Just as a fire needs continual fuel to burn brightly, so too does a relationship require ongoing attention and affection to flourish. In nurturing these bonds, couples can revel in a dynamic and enduring connection that truly celebrates the essence of love.

Romantic Gestures and Surprises

In the vibrant tapestry of a long-term relationship, romantic gestures and surprises act as subtle yet powerful threads that weave passion back into the everyday fabric of life. These small acts of love and thoughtfulness can ignite sparks, often overlooked, breathing fresh warmth into routines that time might have dulled. Imagine the simple delight your partner might experience upon finding a handwritten note tucked under their pillow or the thrill of an unexpected weekend getaway. Gestures like cooking a cherished meal, reliving a first date, or orchestrating an impromptu dance in the living room can transform ordinary moments into extraordinary memories. By embracing creativity and spontaneity, you're not just adding a dash of novelty; you're crafting an ongoing dialogue of love that speaks volumes without uttering a word. These surprises renew affection and remind you both of the fundamental attraction that first brought you together, paving the path to deeper intimacy and a more fulfilling connection.

Planning Date Nights is an art that holds the potential to transform routine evenings into magical escapades, contributing significantly to reigniting passion in long-term relationships. In the rhythm of daily life, where obligations and commitments often take precedence, it's essential to carve out intentional moments to nurture intimacy. Date nights, thoughtfully planned, are powerful tools in your romantic arsenal—each one an opportunity to step away from the mundane and reconnect with your partner.

Start by recognizing that date nights don't have to be grand or lavish to be effective. The key lies in the intention behind them. What matters most is the shared experience and the conscious effort to prioritize your relationship. In the bustle of life, dedicating time to be together can communicate volumes to your partner. It's a silent yet powerful affirmation that amidst all the chaos, the connection you share remains paramount.

When planning a date night, consider the preferences and desires of both you and your partner. It's about crafting an experience that resonates with both of you, allowing shared interests to shine through. Perhaps it's a quiet evening under the stars, a culinary adventure exploring new cuisines, or a spontaneous road trip to a nearby town. The activity itself is secondary to the quality time spent together, fostering closeness and reigniting the passion that brought you together.

Incorporate elements of surprise to keep things fresh and exciting. Surprises, by their nature, spark curiosity and anticipation, which can heighten the emotional connection and deepen the sense of intimacy. This could be as simple as organizing a picnic in a secluded park or scheduling a couple's massage without prior notice. The thrill of the unexpected not only energizes the relationship but also underscores the effort and thoughtfulness invested in planning.

A key component of planning successful date nights is communication. Engage in an open dialogue with your partner about your expectations and experiences. Reflect on past date nights to understand what worked and what didn't, using these insights to plan future outings. This not only ensures that both partners are satisfied but also strengthens communication—a cornerstone of any thriving relationship.

Consider making planning date nights a collaborative effort. Sit down together and brainstorm ideas, allowing creativity to flow from both sides. This partnership in planning can be an enjoyable prelude to the actual date, setting the stage for shared excitement and anticipation. Furthermore, it ensures that the evening caters to both partners' tastes, fostering a sense of equality and mutual enjoyment.

Don't shy away from routine in date nights if that's what feels comforting and intimate. There's beauty in familiarity—some couples find joy in revisiting the place where they had their first date or recreating meals they've enjoyed together in the past. This can evoke nostalgia and remind both partners of the journey they've shared, reinforcing the love and memories that anchor their relationship.

In terms of logistics, simplicity can often be more impactful than complexity. When burdened with intricate plans, the stress of execution might overshadow the joy of the experience. Aim for casual and relaxed outings that allow both partners to unwind and be present with each other. Keep things stress-free and allow for spontaneous changes if that's what the moment calls for.

Another consideration is the frequency of these date nights. While the ideal frequency may vary from couple to couple, finding a regular rhythm is important. Whether it's a weekly commitment or a monthly get-together, the regularity helps in continually nurturing and reinforcing the romantic connection. Remember, the emphasis is on quality, not quantity. Even brief moments can have profound impacts when infused with genuine affection and attention.

Furthermore, planning date nights is an opportunity to explore new aspects of your relationship. Experiment with activities that neither of you has tried before, introducing an element of novelty that can invigorate your connection. This not only adds excitement but can also open new avenues for growth and discovery within the relationship.

In conclusion, date nights are more than just scheduled outings; they are the heartbeats in the symphony of romance that sustain the flame of love in long-term relationships. By infusing creativity, excitement, and intent, these evenings can become cherished rituals that not only rekindle passion but also lay the foundation for deeper intimacy and understanding. As you navigate the journey of love, let each date night be a testament to your commitment, creativity, and eternal desire to keep the spark alive.

Spontaneous Acts of Love can serve as a beacon of warmth, reigniting the passion and connection in long-term relationships. The challenge lies in breaking the monotony that naturally develops over time. Injecting surprise and spontaneity into daily life can combat routine and rekindle romance. Oftentimes, it's the unexpected, heartfelt gestures that cement a couple's bond and remind them of why they fell in love in the first place. Simple, thoughtful actions like leaving a sweet note in your partner's bag or preparing their favorite meal without prompting can speak volumes more than grand declarations.

Our lives are often cluttered with schedules and responsibilities, both professional and personal, that leave little room for spontaneity. Making time to plan an impromptu picnic, a surprise day trip, or an unexpected evening under the stars can create shared memories that deepen the bond between partners. The goal is to express love in a way that resonates with your partner, acknowledges their preferences, and fosters intimacy. These small, sincere gestures act as a reminder that even amidst routine, love continues to be a dynamic, ever-evolving force.

Imagine coming home to a surprise setup of your favorite movie and a cozy blanket fort reminiscent of simpler times. Such unplanned acts of care and attention provide a playful escape from the ordinary, a reset button amidst the whirlwind of everyday obligations. Surprises that tap into nostalgia can be particularly powerful, as they reaffirm the shared history that forms part of the couple's unique tapestry.

Understanding your partner's love language can be pivotal in the realm of spontaneous acts of love. Whether it's words of affirmation, acts of service, receiving gifts, quality time, or physical touch, knowing how your partner feels cherished enables you to tailor your surprises to their unique personality. An unexpected compliment, a spontaneous foot massage after a long day, or an unsolicited act of kindness can foster a deep sense of connection, affirming each partner's commitment to the relationship.

Moreover, spontaneous acts don't always have to be meticulously planned or involve significant effort. Sometimes, simply seizing the moment can lead to memorable exchanges. Catching a beautiful sunset on the way home or dancing in the rain can transform ordinary occurrences into extraordinary experiences. It's these instances that often lead to laughter and joy, reinforcing the whimsical, unpredictable nature of life and love.

However, spontaneity doesn't mean impulsivity without consideration, especially in the context of a relationship. It's about being attuned to your partner's needs and desires. Random acts of love should enhance comfort and understanding, not disrupt it. By being attentive and affectionate without prior prompting or obligation, couples can foster a nurturing environment where love thrives unchecked. It's a delicate balance of understanding boundaries while also embracing the unexpected.

In navigating spontaneity, patience and communication are key. Partners should feel comfortable sharing what surprises make them happy and feel appreciated. Open discussions about desires and dislikes can prevent missteps and ensure both have a fulfilling emotional and romantic experience. After all, true spontaneity and romantic gestures stem from an intimate knowledge of and empathy for each other.

Creating these moments of spontaneity can also be about rediscovering mutual interests and shared activities that have been left aside as life has grown busier. Is there a hobby or interest both partners loved but haven't indulged in for years? Revisiting these shared joys can reignite old passions and spark new connections. Perhaps you both loved painting, hiking, or attending concerts. Arranging a surprise outing can resurrect those neglected passions and provide new avenues for bonding.

Spontaneous acts of love serve as a testament to the strength and evolution of a relationship. They highlight the desire not only to maintain the connection but also to nurture it continually. Through creativity, mindfulness, and genuine affection, couples can keep the spark alive, defying the tendency toward complacency. Such gestures affirm that while love is enduring, it thrives on novelty and surprise.

Ultimately, love in long-term relationships thrives on the balance of stability and surprise. Spontaneous acts emphasize the thrill of the unexpected while reinforcing the profound, unwavering love that binds two souls together. As couples navigate the ebbs and flows of life, these small but impactful gestures can bring joy and reaffirm the dynamic, lively power of love. So, go ahead and embrace the art of spontaneity—every surprise is a brushstroke on the canvas of a shared life.

Chapter 10:
The Role of Mental Health

Mental health plays a crucial role in our intimate relationships, shaping how we connect with our partners and experience desire. Understanding the intricacies of our minds can lead to a more fulfilling and passionate love life. When depression or anxiety creeps in, they can dull the once-vibrant flames of passion, making it vital to address and manage these mental health challenges. Therapy and counseling offer avenues for healing, providing partners with tools to communicate more effectively and develop deeper emotional bonds. Exploring therapy isn't just about solving problems—it's about fostering growth and enhancing intimacy. Different therapeutic options can help uncover underlying issues and offer fresh perspectives, ultimately rejuvenating both individual well-being and relational harmony. By nurturing our mental health, we open the door to rediscovering joy and connection, enriching our romantic interactions in profound and meaningful ways.

Addressing Depression and Libido

Depression is a complex and pervasive mental health challenge that impacts millions worldwide. Often, its grip extends deeper than mood, affecting various facets of life—including intimate relationships. When we talk about libido, or sexual desire, it's crucial to recognize how mental health conditions like depression can directly influence it. Understanding this link allows us to approach the matter with empathy and informed care, focusing on a path to healing and revitalization.

The relationship between depression and libido is intricate and multifaceted. Depression can lead to a decrease in libido due to a variety of factors, including diminished energy levels, reduced self-esteem, and decreased interest in activities that were once pleasurable. This lack of desire is not a reflection of the love or bond shared with a partner but rather a symptom of the broader mental health issue at play. Recognizing this can be both liberating and exceedingly challenging for those experiencing it.

It's not uncommon for a person struggling with depression to feel trapped in a cycle. Depression decreases libido, which can then contribute to feelings of guilt or inadequacy if their partner feels neglected or misunderstands the situation. Open communication becomes vital here. Couples are encouraged to talk candidly about these challenges and support each other through the healing process. Compassionate dialogue can help dispel myths and reduce the shame often associated with a diminished sex drive.

Treating depression is a critical step in restoring libido. Fortunately, multiple treatment options are available, each offering a unique approach to managing and potentially alleviating the symptoms of depression. These can include therapy, medication, lifestyle changes, and holistic practices, all of which can contribute to improved mental health and, consequently, an increased desire for intimacy.

When it comes to therapy, cognitive behavioral therapy (CBT) is particularly effective. It helps individuals recognize and alter negative thought patterns that contribute to feelings of depression. By fostering a change in perception, CBT aims to elevate mood, cultivate a more positive outlook on life, and thereby enhance libido indirectly. Likewise, modalities like acceptance and commitment therapy (ACT) can help individuals focus on living mindfully and embracing their values, encouraging a renewed sense of desire.

Medications, such as antidepressants, can be instrumental in treating depression. However, they can also have side effects that include altering sexual function or decreasing libido. It's essential for individuals to maintain open lines of communication with healthcare providers to address these concerns. Adjustments can be made, whether that involves changing the medication, dosage, or integrating complementary therapies. It's a journey to be navigated collaboratively, with professionals working alongside individuals and their partners.

Incorporating lifestyle changes that promote overall mental well-being can also prove beneficial. Regular physical activity, for example, has been shown to enhance mood, reduce symptoms of depression, and boost libido by increasing endorphin levels. Exercise also provides a sense of accomplishment and enhances body image, which can play a significant role in how one perceives themselves in a relationship.

Additionally, nutrition can play its part in the intricate dance between mental health and libido. A balanced diet rich in essential nutrients supports brain health, leading to improved mood and energy levels. Omega-3 fatty acids, complex carbohydrates, and proteins can positively impact neurotransmitter function, thereby potentially improving both mental health and sexual desire.

Holistic approaches such as mindfulness, meditation, and yoga can be excellent complements to more traditional therapies. These practices promote mental clarity and relaxation while also encouraging individuals to become more attuned to their bodies. By fostering a sense of mindfulness, one can rekindle a sense of curiosity and desire. Partners may consider practicing these activities together, which also strengthens emotional and physical bonds.

Throughout this journey, the underlying theme is connection—both internal and with one's partner. When facing depression and its impact on libido, connection becomes not just a desire but a lifeline. Engaging in intentional time together, cultivating patience, and practicing empathy can keep the river of intimacy flowing, even when it feels obstructed by the rough terrain of mental health challenges.

It's important to remember that every relationship's journey is different. What works for one couple might not work for another. The path to rekindling desire lies in understanding, patience, and the willingness to explore different avenues of healing and connection. By addressing depression with earnest efforts and compassionate communication, the bridge to reclaiming libido and enriching intimacy can be crossed together.

Therapy and Counseling Options

In the journey to enhance libido and deepen intimate connections, therapy and counseling emerge as invaluable resources, embracing both the complexities and beauty of mental health. They offer a tailored approach to each couple, empowering them to navigate emotional hurdles and rejuvenate their passion. Engaging with a therapist can foster a safe space for exploring underlying issues that may dampen desire, be it stress, past trauma, or communication breakdowns. With a variety of therapeutic methods available—from cognitive-behavioral therapy to sex therapy—couples are guided toward understanding and transforming their emotional landscapes. This collaboration not only reignites desire but nurtures a profound bond, aligning mental well-being with the intricate symphony of intimacy. In seeking these paths, couples unlock the potential to cultivate a fulfilling and harmonious relationship, where passion and connection flourish hand in hand.

Types of Therapy can offer a transformative path for those seeking to enhance their intimate connections and reignite passion in their relationships. In navigating the intricate interplay of mental health and desire, different therapeutic approaches provide unique insights and tools that can deepen understanding, foster emotional intimacy, and ultimately enrich one's romantic life. Even though therapy can seem intimidating or unfamiliar, it holds the promise of unraveling the complexities that often stand between partners and the intimacy they seek.

One of the most widely recognized forms of therapy is *Cognitive Behavioral Therapy (CBT)*. It's a structured, goal-oriented approach that helps individuals identify and restructure negative thought patterns that may inhibit libido and intimacy. Often, anxiety, performance pressure, or past traumas can manifest as mental barriers, dampening desire. CBT equips individuals with practical coping strategies, transforming these challenges into opportunities for growth. In doing so, it not only enhances personal well-being but also contributes positively to one's romantic relationships.

On a different note, *Psychodynamic Therapy* delves deeper into the unconscious processes influencing behavior. This method seeks to uncover underlying conflicts that might be impacting a person's ability to connect intimately. By exploring deep-seated emotions and childhood experiences, individuals gain insight into their relational patterns. This self-awareness can lead to profound changes in how one perceives and communicates with a partner, fostering a more open and fulfilling connection.

For couples specifically, *Couples Therapy* becomes a vital resource. It provides a structured environment for partners to communicate openly about their issues, with a mediator to guide the process. Whether dealing with conflicts, miscommunications, or a simple disconnect, couples therapy focuses on enhancing understanding and empathy between partners. By addressing grievances in a safe space, it helps partners collaborate on solutions, thereby strengthening their bond. It's a reminder that relationships, much like any other living entity, require nourishment and attention to thrive.

Sex Therapy, on the other hand, zeroes in on sexual concerns that might be influencing libido. It can cover a range of topics, from sexual dysfunctions to mismatched libidos. By addressing these issues head-on, sex therapy offers a non-judgmental platform for individuals or couples to explore their sexual concerns. The goal is to create a fulfilling and pleasurable sexual relationship, removing any shame or stigma that might hinder sexual expression.

Mindfulness-Based Therapy is another approach gaining popularity for its holistic emphasis on being present. By cultivating mindfulness, individuals learn to savor the moment without distractions, which can enrich intimate experiences. This form of therapy often incorporates techniques like meditation and body awareness to enhance one's connection to their own desires and to their partner's needs. It's about creating an intimacy that extends beyond the physical, nurturing an emotional bond that stands the test of time.

For those who relate to emotional blocks or past traumas affecting their present relationships, *Trauma-Informed Therapy* can be particularly beneficial. Such therapy understands and responds to the aftermath of trauma, offering a pathway to healing that respects the individual's emotional scars. By empowering individuals to reclaim control over their narratives, it aids in rebuilding trust and safety within oneself and with a partner.

The advent of technology has also seen the rise of *Online Therapy*, which offers flexibility and accessibility for those who may find traditional therapy settings challenging. Through virtual sessions, individuals and couples can access professional guidance from the comfort of their homes, making therapy more inclusive and adaptable to modern lifestyles.

In conclusion, the *Types of Therapy* available are multifaceted, each offering a unique lens through which to view and enhance one's intimate relationships. The journey through therapy can illuminate parts of oneself that demand care and attention, part of a broader tapestry woven with threads of understanding, compassion, and love. By embracing therapy, individuals take a proactive step towards a healthier, more passionate relational life, embracing both vulnerability and strength in their quest for deeper connection.

How to Seek Help In our journey towards enhancing intimacy and reigniting passion, addressing our mental health is not only beneficial but necessary. Sometimes, it can be daunting to admit that professional help is required, but recognizing this need is a courageous first step towards a fulfilling love life. If you notice persistent feelings of anxiety, depression, or other emotional barriers that affect your relationship or sexual desire, it's time to seek help. Therapists and counselors offer a safe space to explore these challenges, gain insight, and develop practical strategies to overcome them.

Therapy and counseling can be transformative experiences. They offer a unique opportunity to gain deeper understanding—not just of the self but of one's partner and the dynamics of the relationship as well. There are various types of therapy that cater to different needs, from individual therapy to couples counseling. By discussing goals and preferences with a qualified professional, a tailored approach can be created that addresses specific needs.

Initiating therapy might seem daunting at first, but choosing the right therapist or counselor can ease this process. Begin by researching different therapy modalities such as cognitive-behavioral therapy (CBT) or psychodynamic therapy. Each approach offers different benefits, and finding the right match can make a world of difference.

Consider what resonates with you and what might best address the particular challenges you're facing.

Online therapy platforms have made accessing mental health support more convenient than ever. These platforms offer the flexibility of having sessions from the comfort of your own home and often provide a wider selection of therapists. They're particularly beneficial for those balancing a demanding lifestyle or those who prefer a more private setting. Exploring these options can open up new avenues for support.

Affordability can sometimes be a barrier to seeking help. However, many therapists offer sliding scale fees based on income, and there are community clinics that provide services at reduced rates or even pro bono for those in financial need. It's important not to let financial concerns prevent you from reaching out for the help you need; there are often options available to make therapy accessible.

Building a trusting relationship with your therapist is vital for the therapeutic process to be effective. It's perfectly okay to have introductory sessions with a few different professionals before committing to one. During these sessions, consider how comfortable you feel discussing your intimate concerns and if the therapist's style aligns with your expectations. A strong therapeutic alliance is a foundation for progress and healing.

Once therapy begins, engage fully in the process. Such openness can lead to profound personal growth and enriched relationships. Communication is key; don't hesitate to voice any concerns during your sessions. Therapy is a collaborative effort where your input is crucial to finding the most effective path forward.

In addition to traditional therapy, group therapy or support groups can also be highly beneficial. Sharing experiences in a group setting can provide a sense of community and understanding, proving that you are not alone in your struggles. These groups can be an excellent complement to individual or couples therapy, offering different perspectives and shared experiences that foster resilience and growth.

Remember, seeking therapy does not imply weakness; rather, it demonstrates strength and a commitment to personal and relational growth. It's an investment in oneself and the relationships that matter most. Finding the right help can transform barriers into opportunities for enhanced connections and intimacy.

Ultimately, the decision to seek help is deeply personal and varies from individual to individual. It involves reflecting on your needs and addressing any hesitations head-on. Once you embark on this journey, the potential for personal and relational growth is boundless. Seek help with confidence, knowing that it's a step towards a more intimate and passionate partnership.

Chapter 11:
The Impact of Lifestyle Choices

Our daily choices wield enormous power over our intimate lives, shaping how we connect with our partners. It's a delicate dance where habits like smoking, excessive alcohol, and drug use can dull the vibrancy of desire, creating distances we're often unaware of. However, through conscious lifestyle adjustments, we ignite a beacon of hope and renewal. Imagine a life where choosing fresh, nourishing foods and nurturing your body becomes a catalyst for closeness; where letting go of harmful habits breathes new energy into your relationship. Embracing moderation and seeking positive changes aren't just acts of self-care, but declarations of love for your partner, laying the groundwork for a more fulfilling and passionate connection. Taking steps towards these healthier choices not only enriches individual wellbeing but weaves a richer tapestry of intimacy and satisfaction in your most cherished relationships.

Smoking, Alcohol, and Drug Use

Among the intricate dance of lifestyle choices affecting intimacy, smoking, alcohol, and drug use cast long shadows that can obscure the path to a fulfilling romantic life. These elements, often glamorized and symbolized as tokens of spontaneity and freedom, bear consequences that can stem the flow of desire. When we explore the ties between these habits and libido, we uncover layers of impact that are crucial for any couple striving to rejuvenate their connection.

Cigarette smoking introduces a complex array of chemicals into the bloodstream, which can constrict blood vessels. These effects ripple through the body, adversely affecting circulation. Poor circulation can impair the body's ability to respond sexually. Furthermore, long-term smoking can particularly impact men by contributing to erectile dysfunction. The alluring image of a cigarette between fingers may be tempting, but it subtly undermines the physical foundation of desire.

Quitting smoking can seem daunting, yet it stands as a powerful step toward not only improving one's health but also rekindling the passion with your partner. As the body heals and circulation improves, many find an unexpected resurgence in energy and responsiveness, laying groundwork for rejuvenated experiences of intimacy. This journey requires perseverance, but witnessing the revival of warmth in your relationship offers profound encouragement.

Alcohol, often perceived as a social lubricant, dances a line between slight enhancement and profound hindrance of sexual desire. Its initial effects can lower inhibitions, creating an illusion of heightened sexual interest and confidence. Once alcohol becomes excessive, it can disrupt the body's delicate hormonal balance and impair judgment, leading often to unsatisfying experiences or moments that are difficult to remember or cherish.

Binge drinking can take a toll on emotional and physical intimacy. Alcohol affects the brain's communication pathways, altering mood and behaviors in ways that can erode trust and harmony. For couples to reignite desire while incorporating alcohol, moderation is key. By savoring moments with a single glass to enhance rather than overwhelm a romantic dinner, experiences can maintain their richness without compromising connection.

Recreational drug use introduces another layer of complexity to intimacy. These substances vary widely in their effects; however, they often carry potential to disrupt natural neurotransmitter systems. While usage can lead to initial feelings of euphoria or heightened sensation, it frequently comes at a steep cost to long-term sexual health and relationship dynamics.

For instance, drugs such as cocaine and amphetamines can create an intense and temporary feeling of arousal. Still, habitual use diminishes the brain and body's natural responses to stimuli, leaving a dulled ability to find pleasure in everyday moments of intimacy. Additionally, substance abuse can become a profound source of conflict within a relationship, straining the foundational elements of trust and understanding.

It's essential to approach these habits with a spirit of openness and reflection. Reevaluating the role these substances play in your intimate life involves both partners engaging in honest dialogues. Seeking support from each other and, if necessary, professional resources, becomes paramount in shifting towards healthier lifestyle choices that are conducive to desire.

Exploring alternatives to these habits can also act as a bonding activity. Couples can discover new sources of joy and relaxation that do not compromise their connection. Whether it's exploring mindfulness practices like meditation, enjoying new physical activities together, or indulging in creative or cultural pursuits, these alternatives can catalyze a deeper appreciation for one another.

Embarking on the journey to minimize or eliminate smoking, drinking, and drug use promises not only a return to physical health but a rediscovery of what truly enhances passion between lovers. It's a venture toward not only self-improvement but an expression of care and commitment to sustaining the vitality of your relationship.

By acknowledging the impacts of these substances on libido and intimacy, couples can refocus on nurturing a shared life free from these constraints. Here lies the potential to cartographically re-draw the boundaries of their desire, unclouded by the fog of addiction or habitual indulgence. The path may be challenging, but the rewards—a rekindled romance, enriched connection, and robust desire—are well worth the effort.

Healthy Lifestyle Adjustments

In the dance of intimacy, adopting healthy lifestyle adjustments can be the gentle yet transformative steps that elevate your partnership to new heights. By embracing habits that nurture your overall well-being, you're not just investing in your physical health, but also in the vibrant energy of your intimate life. This journey begins with small, intentional changes that can ripple through your relationship. Prioritizing nourishing foods, engaging in regular exercise, and ensuring a restful sleep can all contribute to a more balanced state of mind and body. As you harmonize these healthy choices, you're likely to notice an enhancement in desire and connection, turning everyday moments into opportunities for deeper bonding. These adjustments are not merely efforts towards a healthy body; they're acts of love, fostering an environment where passion can flourish. Celebrate each step, knowing that by choosing a healthier lifestyle, you're crafting a shared path filled with vitality, joy, and enduring intimacy.

Reducing Harmful Habits is a vital component when discussing the broader topic of lifestyle choices and their impact on libido. Lifestyle habits, often cultivated over the years, can subtly yet significantly influence one's desire and intimate connection with a partner. While some choices may appear minor, their cumulative effect can become apparent when considering overall wellbeing, including sexual health. To truly enhance intimacy and passion, as well as maintain a healthy libido, reducing harmful habits becomes not just beneficial, but essential.

Let's delve into one of the most widespread challenges: smoking. Whether it's cigarettes or other forms of tobacco, these can have severe implications on your health and desire. Smoking impacts circulation, a critical factor in sexual arousal and performance. It also lowers endurance levels, making long-lasting passion challenging. By reducing or ultimately quitting smoking, you open doors to better circulation, increased vitality, and thus heightened libido. It's not just about physical improvements; the boost in confidence from overcoming such an addiction can also feed into a more positive and engaging sexual connection.

Alcohol consumption is another factor that can weigh heavily on intimate desires. While a glass of wine might help set the mood, excessive alcohol can numb the senses, delay reactions, and dampen libido. It's a delicate balance, finding the threshold where alcohol lubricates social interactions without drowning desire. Cutting down on alcohol intake, or moderating it, is an actionable step. This decision not only nurtures physical health but also sharpens mental clarity, enabling a more present and connected partnership experience.

Substance use extends beyond tobacco and alcohol. Drugs, both recreational and prescription-based, can play a dual role in one's sexual health. While some substances might be prescribed with the intent to improve health, others recreationally used can diminish sexual sensitivity and performance. It isn't just about the physical effects; there's an emotional toll that comes with relying on substances, potentially creating a barrier between partners. By reducing dependence on such substances, we cultivate space for genuine connections rooted in sobriety and mutual trust.

Of course, relationships thrive on habits that nurture intimacy rather than hinder it. Lifestyle adjustments often require a shift in routine and priorities. This doesn't mean a complete transformation overnight, but rather a series of small, mindful steps. Consider starting with sleep. Quality sleep is the secret sauce for many aspects of our wellbeing, libido included. Improving sleep hygiene—consistent bedtimes, creating a restful sleeping environment, and reducing screen time before bed—can rejuvenate energy and enhance desire.

Nutrition cannot be overlooked when discussing lifestyle adjustments. Foods laden with sugars and unhealthy fats are common culprits in fostering lethargy and dimming desire. Transitioning to a diet rich in whole foods, vitamins, and essential nutrients not only fuels the body but invigorates a more spirited romantic life. This dietary shift isn't about deprivation but about choosing vitality and connection. Partnering on this journey can further strengthen bonds, as you explore new recipes and share in culinary adventures that are as delightful as they are healthy.

Acknowledging and reducing stress is another impactful lifestyle change. Stress exerts a silent but powerful influence over libido. When tension from work, family obligations, or financial concerns infiltrates, desire inevitably wanes. Incorporating stress-reduction techniques such as mindfulness, exercise, or engaging in hobbies offers a reprieve from everyday pressures, making room for desire to flourish. These practices foster a mental space where love and intimacy can be cultivated without the shadows of stress looming large.

It's also crucial to examine the pace of modern life. The incessant push and pull of a fast-paced lifestyle can inadvertently encourage habits that impair libido. Take time management, for instance. Over-scheduling, while it may yield productivity, can starve your relationship of the time and attention it deserves. By reducing commitments and allowing for downtime, you nurture the quality of your intimate connection. Prioritizing time for yourself and your partner isn't indulgent; it's essential for a thriving relationship.

For some, reducing these negative habits may involve seeking support. Whether it's through professional guidance, like therapy or counseling, or pursuing mutual goals with your partner, the path to transformation is often smoother when not walked alone. Opening channels for honest communication about these habits can illuminate shared intentions and goals, ultimately rejuvenating your partnership.

As you embark on these lifestyle adjustments, remember this not an overnight journey. It's ongoing—a continuous series of choices that move you closer to a healthier, more invigorated connection with your partner. Reducing harmful habits might require effort, yet the rewards—a more passionate, authentic relationship—are well worth it. Herein lies the genuine potential of rekindling desire and cultivating an intensely fulfilling love life.

Promoting Positive Changes Embracing a healthier lifestyle offers more than just physical benefits; it's a catalyst for enhancing intimacy and desire. In a world brimming with distractions and stressors, the subtle ways we treat our bodies have a profound impact on our relationships. By fostering positive lifestyle changes, we create an environment ripe for passion and connection.

Start by building a foundation of awareness. Recognizing the habits that hinder your libido, such as excessive screen time or poor dietary choices, is the first step. Awareness breeds change, and acknowledging these patterns empowers you to make mindful decisions. Instead of dwelling on past habits, focus on the possibilities that new, positive behaviors can bring.

One significant change that benefits both mind and body is integrating regular physical activity into your daily routine. Exercise is known to improve mood, reduce stress, and increase stamina—all key elements to enhancing libido. Activities like yoga not only strengthen the body but also teach mindfulness, creating a deeper connection between partners through shared experiences.

Incorporating a balanced diet is equally vital. Whole foods, rich in essential vitamins and minerals, nourish your body and fuel desire. Transforming meals into opportunities for connection is a powerful shift—cooking together can be an intimate, sensual experience. Share the joy of creating nutritious, delicious dishes that invigorate both body and bonds.

Reducing harmful habits is crucial in this transformative journey. Cutting back on alcohol and quitting smoking can lead to significant improvements in desire and performance. These substances often act as hindrances to sexual health, dampening your ability to form authentic and passionate connections. Embrace moderation, or opt for alternative activities that promote health and well-being.

Positive change isn't just about the physical; it's about creating mental space to nurture your relationship. By practicing relaxation techniques such as meditation or deep breathing exercises, you enhance your emotional resilience. This emotional strength allows you to face challenges with your partner rather than against them, fostering deeper intimacy.

Every small step towards a healthier lifestyle contributes to reigniting passion. Celebrate these changes together, acknowledging each other's progress and encouraging consistency. Cultivating an atmosphere of support and motivation enhances not only individual well-being but also the relationship as a whole.

Furthermore, consider the environment in which you live. A clutter-free, beautifully organized space can have a calming effect, setting the mood for romance. Engage all your senses by using calming scents, soft lighting, and soothing sounds to create an inviting and intimate atmosphere.

The journey of promoting positive changes involves continuous learning and adaptation. Stay curious and open to trying new approaches that support healthier choices. Whether you're diving into a new fitness class or learning about the latest nutritional discoveries, sharing the learning experience strengthens your bond.

Moreover, redefine your relationship with time. Prioritize moments that matter by allocating time to each other without distractions. These intervals serve as sacred escapes from hectic schedules, fostering communication and intimacy. Make time spent together a deliberate and cherished part of your routine.

Remember, this journey is personal and unique to every couple. Encourage conversations about desires and comfort zones to ensure that both partners feel valued and heard. By promoting a safe and understanding environment, you're not only enhancing your relationship; you're building a future filled with love and desire.

Ultimately, the aim is to create a lifestyle that supports a vibrant, intimate partnership. Embracing positive changes, be they diet, exercise, or emotional discipline, prepares the ground for a fulfilling, connected, and passionate life with your partner. Allow these changes to be the gentle push your relationship needs, and watch as intimacy flourishes in unexpected and delightful ways.

Chapter 12:
Hormonal Imbalances and Treatment

In the intricate ballet of intimacy, hormones choreograph some of the most critical moves, subtly yet powerfully influencing libido and desire. Disruptions in this delicate balance can sometimes manifest as frustrations in one's intimate life, creating barriers that seem insurmountable. Understanding hormonal influences is key to unraveling these complexities. Thankfully, the realm of treatment options is as diverse as it is hopeful, offering both medical interventions and natural alternatives. Medical solutions might involve targeted therapies and medications that stabilize hormonal levels, enabling the rekindling of intimacy with newfound vigor. Alternatively, embracing natural methods, such as lifestyle adjustments and herbal remedies, can subtly restore balance in a holistic manner. Each pathway not only opens the door to rejuvenated passion but also reinforces the profound connection partners share, turning potential obstacles into opportunities for deeper understanding and growth.

Understanding Hormonal Influence

Hormones are the silent architects of our desires, weaving through the intricate tapestry of our bodies and influencing our deepest cravings. When we speak of libido, it's crucial to appreciate the role of hormones—tiny chemical messengers that stir feelings of attraction, connection, and fulfillment. Understanding hormonal influence provides insight into how our bodies function and why sometimes the rhythm of passion can sway out of time.

Libido is not a constant and can fluctuate with life's natural ebbs and flows. Hormones like testosterone, estrogen, and progesterone ebb and surge throughout different stages of life, shaping our sexual experiences. For instance, testosterone, often dubbed the "hormone of desire," plays a significant role in stimulating sexual interest in both men and women. A drop in its levels might lead to a decrease in libido, while a surge can ignite a passionate flame.

However, hormones don't exist in a vacuum; their influence is intricately linked with other facets of our health. For example, stress, a common culrprit of reduced libido, can elevate cortisol levels, which can, in turn, dampen sexual desire. This biochemical interplay reveals how our emotional and physical health are intertwined. Therefore, tending to our well-being is as much about nurturing our spirit as it is about maintaining hormonal harmony.

Beyond the biological, there's a deeply sensual and emotional aspect to these changes. Hormonal shifts during puberty, pregnancy, postpartum, and menopause symbolize life's transitions, each stage bringing its own blend of challenges and potential. For instance, pregnancy hormones may fluctuate and enhance sensual experiences for some, yet pose challenges for others. Navigating these shifts requires understanding and compassion, both for oneself and between partners.

The delicate dance of hormones throughout a woman's menstrual cycle showcases another layer of their profound impact. Each phase of the cycle might summon different levels of desire. Awareness of these natural shifts can encourage partners to embrace an ebb and flow, fostering intimacy at varying times of the month. This knowledge empowers couples to recognize and even anticipate changes, transforming potential barriers into stepping stones for deeper connection.

In men, testosterone levels naturally decline with age, which can affect sexual drive. While this might seem like an inevitable decline, it's an opportunity to explore intimacy in new, more profound ways. It's about rediscovering each other in ways that transcend physical passion, focusing on emotional and mental connections that can be equally, if not more, fulfilling.

It's essential to acknowledge that not all hormonal imbalances are naturally occurring. Lifestyle factors such as diet, sleep, and exercise play a notable role in maintaining hormonal health. A nutrient-rich diet supports hormone production and regulation, while regular physical activity promotes balanced levels of hormones, fostering improved libido. Additionally, consistent, restful sleep nurtures the body's recovery and internal balance, providing a foundation for hormonal stability.

While medical therapies are available to treat imbalances, natural alternatives also offer promising solutions. Essential oils, mindfulness practices, and certain herbal supplements can create synergistic effects that invite hormonal tranquility. For some, these holistic approaches blend seamlessly with conventional medicine, creating a personalized path towards restoring vitality and desire.

In understanding hormonal influence, we unlock a world where science meets art—the art of listening to one's body, respecting its signals, and lovingly tending to its needs. Hormones are not mere biological arbiters; they're part of the human experience, resonating deeply with our emotional and psychological states.

As we deepen our understanding, we learn to appreciate the unique journey of each partner and individual. Passion is not a singular note played on repeat but a melody enriched by life's diverse experiences. Honoring hormonal influences allows couples to explore new dynamics within their relationship, embracing change as a gateway to greater intimacy.

No journey is the same, just as no hormonal balance is identical. Patience and kindness are our guiding lights. By holding space for each other's experiences and adapting with grace to shifting hormonal landscapes, couples can reaffirm their partnership—uniting as allies rather than adversaries against the inevitable changes.

Ultimately, the key lies in understanding and embracing the transformative power of hormones. By doing so, we can reignite desire, reinforce connection, and cultivate a more profound, liberated expression of love that spans the spectrum of human experience. This journey leads to not just a rekindling of passion but a renewal of the bonds that tie hearts together in the beauty of shared life.

Treatment Options

When faced with the complex landscape of hormonal imbalances, understanding the variety of treatment options available can light the path to restoring desire and deepening intimacy. Embracing a tailored approach is crucial as what works for one may not necessarily resonate with another. Medical interventions, such as hormone replacement therapies, offer scientifically backed solutions by addressing deficiencies directly at their source. Meanwhile, natural alternatives provide a gentler touch, drawing from nature's pharmacy and incorporating lifestyle adjustments and holistic practices. Collaborating with healthcare professionals ensures a blend of expert guidance and personal preference, offering a roadmap that respects both physiological needs and emotional well-being. It empowers couples to rediscover harmony in their desires, coupling scientific knowledge with the art of personalized care. As these interventions work often quietly and behind the scenes, they enable partners to focus more fully on nurturing their intimate connections with renewed vigor and passion.

Medical Interventions have emerged as a beacon of hope in the realm of hormonal imbalances and their treatment, particularly when it comes to enhancing libido and fostering intimate connections. In our exploration of treatment options, we'll delve into how medical science can assist in the delicate dance of hormones, which often holds the key to a vibrant love life. For many, understanding these interventions can be transformative, offering a pathway to not only improved physical health but also a deeper emotional connection with one's partner.

Hormones play a critical role in sexual desire, with testosterone, estrogen, and progesterone being the main players. When these hormones are out of balance, it can lead to a decrease in libido, mood swings, and even physical changes that affect intimacy. Medical interventions often begin with a comprehensive evaluation by healthcare professionals, who may use blood tests to assess hormone levels. This diagnostic step is crucial, as it informs the specific type of treatment needed.

Testosterone replacement therapy (TRT) is one of the more common medical treatments for low libido, particularly in men. Low testosterone can lead to decreased sexual desire, erectile dysfunction, and loss of energy. Through TRT, testosterone levels are brought back to their optimal range, often resulting in improved libido, mood, and energy levels. Various forms of TRT are available, including injections, patches, gels, and implants, allowing for personalized treatment plans.

For women, hormone replacement therapy (HRT) addresses symptoms related to menopause, such as a decrease in libido and vaginal dryness. HRT typically involves combinations of estrogen and progesterone to alleviate these symptoms, thus enhancing sexual desire and comfort. However, HRT is not without its potential risks, and the decision to undergo this treatment requires careful consideration and discussion with a healthcare provider to weigh its benefits against possible side effects.

Besides hormonal therapies, contraceptive options such as the pill, patch, ring, or injections can sometimes negatively impact libido due to their hormonal nature. For those experiencing reduced sexual desire as a side effect of contraception, a change in the method or type of contraceptive may be advised. This is another area where medical guidance is invaluable, helping patients find a balance that supports both reproductive health and sexual satisfaction.

Pharmacological interventions extend beyond hormone replacement. Medications such as phosphodiesterase type 5 (PDE5) inhibitors, including sildenafil (Viagra) and tadalafil (Cialis), are commonly prescribed to tackle erectile dysfunction, a significant barrier to satisfying sexual experiences. By improving blood flow and facilitating erections, these medications can help rekindle passion and intimacy for affected individuals.

Interestingly, the field of sexual medicine is continually evolving, with new research and treatments emerging. For instance, oxytocin, often dubbed the "love hormone," is being studied for its potential role in enhancing the emotional connection between partners and increasing sexual desire. Although still in its nascent stages, oxytocin-based treatments could open new avenues for those seeking to enhance their intimate lives through medical interventions.

Moreover, medical interventions aren't just about taking medications or undergoing hormone therapy. Lifestyle modifications often serve as complementary strategies. Medical professionals may recommend changes in diet, exercise, and stress management as part of a holistic approach to treating hormonal imbalances. These lifestyle changes can amplify the effects of medical treatments, leading to a more robust and sustained improvement in libido.

In some cases, underlying medical conditions such as diabetes, thyroid disorders, or depression can contribute to hormonal imbalances and reduced libido. Treating these conditions with the appropriate medical interventions can indirectly restore hormonal balance and improve sexual desire. Therefore, a comprehensive medical evaluation is essential to identify and address any such underlying issues.

Counseling and psychosexual therapy can also be considered a form of medical intervention. These therapies focus on addressing the psychological aspects of low libido, which often accompany or even cause hormonal imbalances. By working through emotional blocks, anxiety, or relationship issues with a trained professional, individuals can achieve significant improvements in their intimate relationships, complementing the effects of medical treatments.

Lastly, it's vital for individuals and couples to communicate openly with healthcare providers about their needs and concerns regarding intimacy and libido. This communication ensures that medical interventions are tailored to the individual's unique circumstances, maximizing their effectiveness and fostering a more fulfilling and passionate intimate life. Adopting a collaborative approach between medical professionals and individuals can lead to the best outcomes in treating hormonal imbalances and enhancing desire.

Natural Alternatives offer a gentle yet effective pathway to addressing hormonal imbalances, inviting harmony and vitality back into your intimate life. In our quest to enhance libido and deepen connections, it's crucial to consider these remedies as part of your holistic approach to wellness. They seamlessly intertwine age-old wisdom with modern life, providing options for those who seek to harness nature's bounty in their pursuit of love and passion.

Herbal remedies have a long history of use in balancing hormones and enhancing sexual health. Maca root, often heralded as a "superfood," stands out for its ability to boost energy and libido. Originating from the Peruvian Andes, it not only supports hormonal equilibrium but also fosters increased stamina and vitality. Another potent herb is Tribulus terrestris, known for its capacity to enhance desire by stimulating androgen receptors in the brain. These botanical allies work synergistically with your body's natural processes, making them a preferred choice for many.

Essential oils are another way to incorporate nature's offerings into your life. The aromatic properties of oils like clary sage and geranium can influence your mood and help balance hormones. They're typically used in aromatherapy, known for creating a relaxing environment that can alleviate stress and improve libido. A simple yet effective practice is to add a few drops of these oils to a warm bath or diffuser, turning ordinary spaces into sanctuaries of peace and connection.

Diet also plays a powerful role in natural hormone regulation. Foods rich in omega-3 fatty acids, such as flaxseeds and walnuts, support hormone production and promote overall health. These fats are essential for maintaining optimal function of the endocrine system. Additionally, incorporating zinc-rich foods like pumpkin seeds and chickpeas can help balance hormones by playing a crucial role in hormone synthesis.

In the delicate dance of hormones, lifestyle adjustments serve as both a stage and a backdrop. The practice of yoga has become an integral way to maintain hormonal harmony. Through a series of specific poses and breathing techniques, yoga aids in reducing stress—a known disruptor of hormone levels. It encourages mindfulness, allowing couples to be present and connected both on and off the mat. The gentle stretching and focused breathing promote circulation and relaxation, which are key to enhancing one's libido.

Integrating these natural alternatives into your daily routine doesn't require an overhaul of your lifestyle; instead, it invites a mindful shift toward using nature's tools to bolster both your physical and emotional well-being. As modern science continues to validate these age-old practices, it becomes increasingly clear that they offer viable pathways to not just balance but flourishing.

When contemplating the inclusion of natural remedies, it's essential to approach them with patience and openness. Unlike the rapid results promised by pharmaceutical interventions, natural alternatives often require time to weave their magic, encouraging a reconnection with one's body and desires. This gentle unfolding can be a transformative experience, deepening intimacy in relationships and nurturing a sense of self-awareness and empowerment.

A consideration for those venturing into this natural territory is self-education—understanding the optimal dosages and applications of herbal supplements and dietary adjustments. Consulting with a healthcare provider or a professional herbalist can ensure that these natural interventions are both safe and suited to individual needs.

In embracing natural alternatives, you become more attuned to the rhythms of your own body and the cycles of nature. This consciousness assists in creating a holistic and enriched intimate experience, one where both partners benefit not just from physical closeness but a shared journey of discovery and wellness.

Ultimately, the path of natural alternatives is not just about treating symptoms of hormonal imbalance; it's about nurturing a lifestyle that promotes balance at every level. By choosing these natural methods, you're not only addressing immediate concerns but cultivating a foundation for healthier relationships—relationships built on understanding, patience, and mutual growth.

As you continue exploring the intimate dance of hormones and desires, remember that each of these natural alternatives offers a step closer to achieving the fulfillment and vibrant connection you seek. May this exploration inspire a deeper appreciation for the delicate balance of nature and the powerful potential it holds to transform your love life from within.

Chapter 13:
Intimate Conversations with Experts

In "Intimate Conversations with Experts," we explore the invaluable insights offered by renowned sex therapists and real-life couples who've successfully navigated the complexities of desire and intimacy. Through engaging dialogues and shared experiences, these experts reveal strategies that empower couples to renew their passion and deepen their connections. By understanding diverse perspectives and learning from others' journeys, readers can glean practical advice and inspiration. Key takeaways include recognizing the power of empathy, the significance of maintaining open channels of communication, and the necessity of continual growth in relationships. These stories don't just provide solutions; they ignite the spark necessary to embark on a fulfilling and transformative journey of love and connection.

Interviews with Sex Therapists

In the realm of intimate relationships, understanding your desires and passions is crucial. But sometimes, untangling the complex web of personal and shared experiences that shape libido can be daunting. Enter sex therapists—experts who bridge the gap between scientific understanding and emotional insight. These professionals bring a wealth of knowledge from years spent helping couples and individuals navigate the intricate dance of desire. Through their work, they offer invaluable wisdom on how to reignite the flame and sustain it through the inevitable changes life throws your way.

One of the remarkable aspects of discussing intimacy with sex therapists is how personalized their advice often becomes. No two people are the same, and these experts honor that individuality. They approach each client with the understanding that what enhances pleasure for one might not work for another. This nuanced perspective allows them to guide individuals on a path that fits their unique needs and experiences. From helping couples reconnect emotionally to offering practical exercises that elevate physical intimacy, their insights cover a broad spectrum of intimate challenges and solutions.

In conversations with these therapists, a common theme emerges: communication. It's no surprise that open dialogue is a cornerstone of successful relationships, but its role in enhancing sexual intimacy is often understated. By fostering an environment where both partners feel safe and heard, couples can explore their desires more freely. Therapists encourage a dynamic exchange of thoughts and feelings, where vulnerability is not seen as a weakness but as a strength—one that opens doors to deeper connections. Techniques such as active listening and expressing needs without judgment foster this open dialogue, making room for growth and intimacy.

Furthermore, sex therapists emphasize the importance of empathy. The ability to step into your partner's shoes, to understand their desires and fears, can be transformative. This empathetic approach isn't just about acknowledging feelings—it involves actively engaging with them in a way that makes both partners feel cherished and valued. When both individuals in a relationship can practice empathy, it's not just the sexual connection that thrives; the overall bond becomes stronger and more resilient.

Another integral piece of advice from sex therapists revolves around overcoming common barriers to desire. Stress, everyday obligations, and even self-doubt can take a toll on libido. The therapists we interviewed suggested a variety of methods to tackle these hurdles. Mindfulness techniques, such as meditation and deep-breathing exercises, help in reducing stress by bringing a sense of calmness and presence. Stress, being one of the most common hindrances in intimacy, often requires consistent management to unravel its hold on desire.

Therapists also suggest viewing intimacy as a series of explorations rather than obligations. By approaching it as an adventure, couples can break free from routine and discover new facets of their connection. Whether through trying novel experiences or simply changing the time and place of intimate encounters, small shifts can lead to big changes in how partners perceive and engage with each other. The idea is to make the journey towards intimacy as enriching as the destination itself.

In these interviews, therapists offer a refreshing take on handling physical changes and aging bodies, often a source of anxiety for many. Aging is a natural part of life, and rather than being seen as a decline, it can be embraced as an opportunity to explore new avenues of intimacy. Emphasizing the importance of body acceptance, therapists encourage couples to discover what feels good now, rather than lamenting what once was. This approach can transform aging from a source of insecurity to a celebration of a life well-experienced, setting a stage where sensuality can continue to bloom.

Many therapists highlight the power of touch and sensuality as fundamental to maintaining intimate connections. The art of sensual massage, for instance, is repeatedly mentioned as a way to reconnect physically and emotionally. Such practices allow partners to express affection and build physical closeness without the pressure of expectation. By focusing on the sensory experiences—how a touch feels, the scent of a favorite lotion, or the warmth of skin against skin—partners can deepen their bond and enhance their corporeal understanding of one another.

Ultimately, the collective insights from sex therapists underscore the importance of recognizing and embracing change. Relationships, like people, evolve. What worked in the past may not be effective now, and that's okay. The key is to keep learning about each other and to be open to trying new things. Such adaptability and willingness to grow together can reignite passion and strengthen intimacy, no matter how long the relationship has been.

In conclusion, interviews with sex therapists offer an enlightening window into the heart of intimacy. Through their guidance, they provide practical advice and emotionally resonant strategies that demystify the many components of desire. They don't just address the challenges; they reveal the beauty and potential that lie in truly understanding and nurturing one's intimate connection. Armed with their expertise, couples are better equipped to navigate the ever-changing landscape of desire, fostering a love that's vibrant and fulfilling.

Real-Life Success Stories

Within the tapestry of human relationships, stories of rekindled passion and deep connection abound, offering a beacon of hope and a guide for others on similar journeys. Take, for instance, Sarah and Tom, who found themselves in a rut after a decade of marriage. Through transformative conversations with an intimacy coach, they discovered the power of empathy and vulnerability, unlocking a newfound emotional closeness that reignited their desire for one another. Then there's Clara and Michael, a couple who revitalized their bond by embracing novel experiences together—melding the thrill of adventure with emotional intimacy, creating an unbreakable foundation of love. These narratives illuminate the path towards a fulfilled and vibrant love life, demonstrating that with determination and the right guidance, any couple can rediscover joy and intimacy.

Each success story reinforces the book's central theme: that with commitment and understanding, one can rejuvenate their relationship and nurture a deeply satisfying connection.

Lessons Learned from the transformative journey through "Real-Life Success Stories" offer a tapestry of insights into the myriad ways individuals and couples have revitalized their libidos and deepened their intimate bonds. The narratives compiled not only highlight the unique paths taken but also underline some universal truths about human connection and desire.

One of the most consistent lessons found across these stories is the power of vulnerability. Couples who dared to openly share their desires, fears, and insecurities often found themselves more deeply connected than ever before. This sharing isn't merely about verbal exchange; it's an emotional and psychological baring of the soul. For many of these couples, acknowledging their need for emotional safety was a turning point—a segue into an openness that cultivated a deeper intimacy. In these stories, embracing vulnerability isn't portrayed as a weakness but as a cornerstone for building durable and passionate relationships.

Moreover, the impact of small, consistent efforts stands out as a significant takeaway. Rather than focusing on grand gestures or seismic shifts, many found success through regular acts of love and care. Whether it was carving out time for weekly date nights, leaving simple love notes, or embracing daily rituals of physical affection, these small actions accumulated over time to reinforce their connection. This gentle persistence illustrates how nurturing desire doesn't always require drastic measures but can blossom through everyday attentiveness and kindness.

Another pivotal lesson is the role of adaptability and willingness to change. Many couples recounted how they had to confront preconceived notions about what intimacy should look like at different stages in their lives. Adapting to life events such as the arrival of children, career changes, or health challenges required open dialogue and flexibility in approach. Those who thrived in maintaining an intimate connection often did so by refusing to cling rigidly to past dynamics, instead allowing their relationships to evolve organically in response to new circumstances.

Furthermore, the tales of triumph over adversity reveal that challenges, when navigated together, can often act as catalysts for deeper connection. Several couples described how facing difficulties like illness, mental health issues, or financial stress tested their bonds but ultimately strengthened their resilience and empathy for each other. These experiences emphasized the necessity of support networks and the importance of seeking help when needed, be it through counseling, therapy, or community groups.

Indeed, communication emerged as a recurring theme. However, the lessons from these stories delve deeply into the nuance of true communicative connection. It's not just about speaking; it's about ensuring both sides feel heard and understood. Techniques like active listening and non-verbal communication played vital roles in bridging gaps and fostering a sense of mutual respect and appreciation. The real-life examples highlighted that effective communication is a skill to be honed and cherished, pivotal to maintaining intimacy.

Attention to individual well-being also surfaced frequently as a critical component. There was a clear recognition that a fulfilling sexual relationship is deeply intertwined with the physical and mental health of both partners. Various narratives shared experiences of undergoing personal transformations through exercise, nutrition, mindfulness practices, or therapy, underscoring the importance of personal growth alongside relational growth.

Finally, these stories collectively impart an enduring truth: the nature of desire is as varied and unique as the individuals themselves.

What rekindles passion for one couple might differ entirely for another. Embracing this diversity and exploring it with curiosity, empathy, and mutual understanding can lead to more fulfilling connections than rigidly trying to apply a one-size-fits-all solution. This understanding also extends to recognizing and respecting the ebbs and flows that naturally occur in long-term relationships.

In summarizing "Lessons Learned" from these real-life success stories, one can't help but feel motivated and inspired. They invite all who read to take a closer look at their connections and encourage the belief that, with effort, empathy, and a willingness to explore and adapt, a deeply satisfying and intimate partnership is within reach. The path to reigniting passion and deepening intimacy is indeed a journey, and these stories serve as trusted guides illuminating the way forward.

Tips from Couples often reveal that the journey toward enhancing libido and deepening a connection isn't just about harnessing expert knowledge, but also about real-life applications of that wisdom. Couples who have successfully navigated challenges in their intimate lives often have invaluable insights that transcend the theoretical. Their stories illuminate pathways that others can follow, offering hope and practical advice that comes from lived experience. These shared anecdotes demonstrate that while each couple's journey is unique, there are common threads that can inspire and guide others on similar paths.

One couple shared that the ritual of expressing gratitude daily became a cornerstone of their relationship. In the midst of busy schedules and life's inevitable stresses, they took a moment each night to share one thing they appreciated about their partner. It was not a grandiose action but a simple, consistent gesture that fostered affection and connection. This practice didn't eradicate life's pressures, but it certainly helped them to keep sight of the love and positivity even when challenges arose.

Another lesson imparted by couples revolves around the power of intentional time together. In a world that seems to demand constant distraction, carving out intentional, undisturbed time can be a formidable challenge. Yet, those who've embraced this often describe transformative experiences. One pair recounted how a weekend technology detox rekindled their connection, allowing for uninhibited conversations and rediscovery of shared interests. They described it as allowing space for spontaneity—a space that had been previously occupied by screens and notifications.

Couples often emphasize the importance of communication that goes beyond words. This includes understanding and respecting each other's non-verbal cues. One couple found that simply becoming more attuned to each other's body language and subtle signals led to a significant boost in intimacy. By recognizing these cues, they were better able to anticipate each other's needs and desires, fostering a deeper understanding and closeness.

The element of surprise and excitement is another theme that emerges from many success stories. Introducing novelty or revisiting past pleasurable experiences can act as powerful reminders of shared joy. A couple spoke about re-creating their first date—something they'd initially brushed off as clichéd but ultimately found to be a delightful journey down memory lane. It reignited a spark that reminded them of the thrill of early romance, yet it was infused with the depth of years spent together.

Furthermore, the concept of vulnerability cannot be overstated. Couples who report thriving intimate lives often mention a willingness to be vulnerable, even when it feels uncomfortable. One striking account involved a couple who revisited past misunderstandings and hurts through open dialogue and empathy, rather than avoidance. This allowed them to mend old wounds and build a stronger, more resilient foundation for mutual trust and passion.

The act of shared goal-setting, whether in lifestyle changes or personal growth, also proves to be a powerful booster of intimacy. Couples who embark on new challenges together—be it a fitness journey or learning a new hobby—often find that their shared experiences enhance their emotional and physical connection. Setting a joint goal gave one couple a sense of partnership and purpose, turning what could have been routine interactions into sources of encouragement and support.

Many partners highlight the benefit of integrating playful activities into their relationship. One pair mentioned implementing a regular "play date" where they explored fun activities together without any real agenda. The lightheartedness often led to laughter which, scientifically speaking, promotes the release of endorphins, bolstering a sense of happiness and contentment. This simple concept can breathe new life into a relationship that has grown accustomed to routine.

One can't ignore the importance of prioritizing physical affection. Whether it's a lingering hug, a spontaneous kiss, or a gentle touch when passing each other, small gestures of affection often serve as the unspoken language of love. Couples frequently mention how these small acts of physical intimacy can build up to a greater sense of emotional connection, breaking down barriers and fostering closeness.

Finally, couples also share that empathy and compassion go a long way. Understanding that each partner's libido may ebb and flow for various reasons—be it stress, health, or emotional turmoil—creates a patient and supportive environment. Real-life stories reinforce that acknowledging these fluctuations without judgment or frustration helps to maintain a balance of respect and desire, paving the way to a more fulfilling intimate relationship.

While these tips from couples offer insightful strategies, they collectively underscore a common theme: intimacy requires nurturing. Just as a garden needs attention to bloom, so does a relationship in which both partners invest time, attention, and love. Whatever path one might choose, these stories remind us that the pursuit of passion and connection is as much about the journey as it is about the destination.

Chapter 14:
The Role of Technology in
Modern Relationships

In today's digital age, technology weaves itself through the fabric of our relationships, offering both opportunities and challenges for enhancing intimacy and connection. With digital communication tools becoming an integral part of our lives, couples have endless avenues to express affection and maintain closeness, no matter the distance. Yet, as screens and devices dominate our waking hours, the key lies in finding a delicate balance that nurtures emotional bonds while avoiding the distractions that can erode them. Carefully managing screen time and being intentional about tech-free moments allows for a deeper, more meaningful engagement with loved ones. By integrating thoughtful digital practices, partners can leverage technology not only to bridge gaps but also to build a foundation of intimacy that supports a fulfilling, passionate relationship. Ultimately, the way we use technology can either enrich or hinder our journey toward a more profound connection, making conscious choices and shared intentions vital to harmonizing modern tools with timeless romance.

Digital Communication Tools

As we navigate the digital age, our relationships have been profoundly shaped by the tools at our disposal. Digital communication tools offer pathways to intimacy and connection that redefine how we interact with our partners. Whether separated by mere blocks or vast oceans, modern technology allows lovers to share in each other's lives like never before. Imagine a couple where one partner is on a business trip; a quick video call before bed can bring a sense of togetherness, even when apart. Technology bridges physical gaps, allowing emotional bonds to stay strong. Yet, like all tools, their impact depends on how we use them, inviting us to be intentional and mindful in our interactions.

Video calls, text messages, and social media platforms have become staples in staying connected. These tools provide an immediacy to communication that can bolster intimacy, making partners more accessible to one another. At times, a simple text message can convey affection and affirmation instantly, a digital whisper of words that say, "I'm thinking of you." This continuous line of communication can nurture a relationship, preventing the feeling of being unnoticed or uncared for. But it's essential to balance digital presence with genuine interaction, ensuring these tools supplement rather than substitute the richness of face-to-face connection.

Emojis and GIFs have silently crept into everyday conversations, adding a visual layer that textual communication lacks. A heart emoji or a playful GIF can express sentiments that often transcend the barriers of language. They've become modern-day hieroglyphs, bridging the gap between written words and emotional expression, allowing couples to communicate playfully and succinctly. It's worth considering how a well-timed emoji can lighten the mood or diffuse tension, artfully turning potential conflict into a shared smile.

In long-distance relationships, digital communication tools become lifelines. Couples are finding innovative ways to feel close, utilizing these tools to bridge the distance. From virtual dinners via Zoom to shared playlists that synchronize moods, technology provides space for shared experiences. For partners separated by miles, these tools don't merely allow communication—they provide a stage for moments to be lived together apart. An unexpected video call during lunch or sharing a song that reminds one of the other can become cherished rituals.

Yet, the flip side of digital immersion exists, too. There lies a danger of allowing screens to erect barriers, with constant notifications pulling attention away from present moments. It's crucial to navigate these distractions mindfully, consciously deciding when to unplug. Couples can benefit from setting boundaries around technology, such as designated device-free times or agreed-upon screen use guidelines. Balancing technology with presence can enhance intimacy, ensuring that digital communication enhances rather than detracts from real-world connection.

Privacy and trust are other dimensions shaped by digital tools. As these technologies evolve, they raise questions about boundaries and security. Sharing passwords or location data might seem like conveniences, but they also require trust and understanding. It's important to have candid discussions about comfort levels and expectations regarding digital transparency. These conversations build trust and establish a shared foundation, allowing each partner to feel respected and valued.

Online dating platforms epitomize the intersection of technology and relationships, opening doors to connections once limited by geography or circumstance. While many find their partners through these platforms, it's necessary to maintain awareness of the role technology plays in shaping perceptions. Authenticity in digital spaces is crucial, encouraging users to present true selves rather than curated facades. For those seeking to deepen intimacy, honesty from the beginning lays the groundwork for meaningful connections.

While the benefits of digital communication tools are manifold, the importance of presence—both digital and physical—can't be understated. Facetime isn't just about seeing but being with one another. The heartbeat of a relationship can echo within these digital landscapes, but it requires intention and attention. Embracing vulnerability in this realm involves a willingness to share openly, crafting intimate conversations that go beyond the superficial to stir the depths of connection.

As we champion these tools for enhancing our relationships, it's equally important to remember their role as augmenters, not replacements for physical touch and face-to-face connection. Technology should be the bridge between moments, not the sole framework for a relationship. Prioritizing shared activities, date nights, and tangible interactions, alongside digital communication, ensures a balanced nurturing of intimacy, weaving both worlds together seamlessly.

The world of digital communication is ever-evolving, promising new ways to connect and communicate. From emerging technologies like virtual reality call experiences to digital journals that couples can create together, the landscape is both exciting and promising. Embracing this with curiosity and care allows couples to thrive, fostering an environment that respects tradition while celebrating innovation. After all, these tools are not just about efficiency—they're about extending the depth, breadth, and joy of sharing our lives with the ones we love.

Managing Screen Time

In today's digital age, balancing screen time with intimacy can be a challenge that requires intentional effort and awareness. As partners seek to enhance their intimate connections, the omnipresence of screens—from smartphones to laptops—can inadvertently create barriers to genuine interaction and disrupt the natural flow of desire. It's crucial to establish boundaries around technology use, allowing couples to carve out sacred spaces for undistracted, face-to-face engagement. By setting specific times to unplug and fostering environments where technology takes a backseat, partners can cultivate a stronger emotional connection and enhance their physical intimacy. The key lies in transforming potential distractions into opportunities for presence and connection, inviting spontaneity and deepening the shared experiences without the glow of screens overshadowing the glow of love. Through these deliberate choices, couples can rediscover the romance and excitement that fuels their passion.

Balancing Technology with Intimacy can feel like walking a tightrope, especially in an era where screens accompany us everywhere. As couples, the challenge lies in recognizing how devices can both connect and divide us. While technology offers avenues for maintaining connection when physically apart, it can unintentionally create emotional chasms when we're physically together. Finding a balance between our digital lives and intimate relationships is crucial, especially when seeking to deepen our connections and enhance our libido.

The allure of a quick scroll through social media or the immediate gratification of notifications can be hard to resist. Yet, every notification ping can disrupt the flow of intimacy, acting as an invisible barrier between partners. It's not just about the time spent on gadgets—it's the quality of time sacrificed. Studies suggest that even the mere presence of a phone can diminish empathy and connection during conversations. So, where do we draw the line? It's about setting boundaries and being intentional with our tech habits. A simple yet powerful practice is to designate tech-free zones or times, such as during meals or an hour before bed, to foster genuine interaction.

But how do we effectively manage our screen time without feeling deprived or simply swapping one habit for another? It begins with awareness and mutual agreement. Partners can collaborate on creating a tech contract, outlining specific rules around screen usage. This agreement can be a couple's manifesto, turning screen time management into a shared goal. By establishing clear rules, like putting phones to bed at a certain hour or keeping devices out of the bedroom, couples can ensure that time spent together remains undisturbed.

Moreover, reclaiming moments for intimacy doesn't always require grand gestures. Sometimes, the little efforts make the most significant difference. Consider the power of a shared playlist or watching a series together consciously, where both engage actively, discussing and interacting rather than passively watching. Through these shared experiences, couples can cultivate a sense of togetherness, transforming technology from a potential divider into a bridge.

Furthermore, it's essential to recognize the different ways technology can be used not just to reconnect with your partner, but to rekindle passion. Apps designed for couples, focusing on enhancing intimacy and fostering communication, can offer a fresh perspective. Interactive features, like joint journaling or shared goals, can provide a playful yet profound avenue for understanding and affirming each other's desires.

While technology offers tremendous benefits, it can also mask deeper issues if not addressed with mindfulness. Often when individuals gravitate towards excessive screen time, it's a symptom rather than the root cause of intimacy barriers. It's crucial to reflect on underlying emotions. Are you using digital escapism to avoid uncomfortable discussions or unaddressed feelings? These questions, while difficult, open the door to meaningful conversations and vulnerability, laying the foundation for deeper connections.

Commitment to balancing tech and intimacy requires consistent effort and reflection. Frequent check-ins with your partner about how technology affects your relationship can offer invaluable insights. These discussions don't have to be formal; they can be spontaneous chats over coffee or during a weekend stroll. The goal is to maintain a continuous conversation about mutual needs and adjustments, ensuring neither partner feels secondary to a device.

In the end, the goal isn't to vilify technology or to portray it as an enemy of intimacy. Instead, it's to harness its potential meaningfully, allowing it to enhance rather than hinder the relationship. As we navigate the complexities of our tech-saturated world, let's remember that behind every screen is a warm, beating heart longing for genuine connection. By consciously managing our screen times, we can create space for spontaneity, passion, and profound intimacy to enter and expand within our relationships.

Avoiding Distractions: In the age of constant connectivity, the allure of our digital devices can often pull us away from the people who matter most. As we navigate the myriad ways in which technology affects modern relationships, it's crucial to recognize and minimize these distractions, especially when striving to manage screen time and deepen intimacy.

The irony of technology is that while it promises connection, it can easily generate distance. How often have you glanced at your partner only to see their face illuminated by the glow of a smartphone? This omnipresent distraction isn't merely a social inconvenience; it can have profound effects on intimacy and desire. Relationships thrive on attention and presence. When a screen perpetually intrudes, it hampers the capacity to engage fully with one's partner, diminishing the depth of emotional and physical connections.

Imagine a couple on a supposed 'date night,' both swiping through social media feeds instead of sharing dreams or memories. It's easy to fall into the trap of digital multitasking, convincing ourselves that we're still 'together,' but are we truly present? Using technology consciously and setting boundaries isn't about eliminating it from your lives; it's about enhancing your quality time and connection. By consciously unplugging, even for just a few hours, we invite more space for passion, creativity, and understanding.

In practical terms, avoiding distractions starts with creating digital-free zones and times. Consider setting a 'no devices' rule during meals. Yes, the world might be a notification away, but dedicating uninterrupted time to each other fosters an atmosphere of openness where communication flourishes. It's this kind of deliberate practice that nurtures desire—it tells your partner, "I see you, and you are worth my undivided attention."

It's not just about limiting digital interaction; it's about replacing it with activities that enhance connection. Could you engage in a shared activity that requires mutual focus and effort? Cooking, playing a game, or walking together without digital interference can serve as anchors of enduring connection. They create shared experiences that nurture intimacy far better than scrolling through separate screens ever could.

When technology becomes intrusive, it's often up to the couple to reclaim their space. Establishing mindful technology use pathways can be transformative. Instead of checking emails before bed, create a winding-down ritual that includes reading together or discussing the highs and lows of the day. Such practices not only foster closeness but also prime your senses for a more intimate connection.

If breaking free from the digital vortex feels overwhelming, begin with small changes. Identify patterns and contexts where technology most disrupts your bond, and take incremental steps to alter them. Perhaps it's a simple 'bedroom curfew' for devices or a commitment to not use phones at certain times on weekends. In doing so, you'll gradually foster a habit of being more emotionally available to each other.

The distractions we face aren't merely the fault of technology; they stem from how we choose to interact with it. Mindful choices about when and how we use technology can rekindle intimacy and reinforce the partnership's foundation. It's about establishing habits that prioritize the relationship over the digital world, elevating the importance of personal interaction.

When you look back in years to come, you likely won't remember the social media posts you liked or the emails you sent late at night. What's most memorable are the countless moments spent building and reinforcing love anew—moments free from the impingement of screens. By minimizing digital distractions, you open a world where passion and desire can flourish naturally and uninterrupted.

Focusing on the essence of the relationship rather than the peripheral noise sharpens the clarity of your connection. In such moments, the hum of daily routine fades, allowing the symphony of love and desire to take center stage. Recognizing the impact of distractions empowers you to cultivate pathways back to one another, nurturing a realm where technology enhances rather than diminishes your connection.

In conclusion, avoiding distractions is a critical aspect of managing screen time well. Embracing this challenge opens the door to a deeper, more meaningful relationship where the presence is the gift you both offer each other. It's not only about looking up from the screen but also reaching out to what really matters—each other.

Chapter 15:
Enhancing Libido in Different Stages of Life

As we navigate through the various stages of life, our libido is subject to change, reflecting the unique demands and dynamics of each phase. In young adulthood, where energy brims and curiosity thrives, desire often comes naturally, driven by exploration and new experiences. However, as the journey transitions into parenthood, the focus may shift, presenting challenges in maintaining intimacy amidst the demands of family life. It's essential to carve out time for each other, creating small rituals or moments where passion can flourish despite the chaos. Embracing these changes with openness and adaptability is crucial. Approach each stage with the understanding that intimacy is not a static entity but a continually evolving connection that, with care and attention, can deepen over time, enhancing both the emotional and physical bonds shared with your partner.

Young Adulthood and Desire

Young adulthood is a vibrant phase of life, characterized by exploration, discovery, and intense desire. It's a time when many individuals are embracing new experiences, building their identities, and learning about themselves and others in profound ways. The quest to enhance libido during this period is often intertwined with a journey of self-discovery and emotional growth.

In the realm of desire, young adults might find themselves experiencing an intense and fluctuating libido. This can be attributed to a combination of biological, psychological, and social factors. The hormonal shifts that occur at this stage of life are often responsible for the high levels of energy and arousal, making this a prime time for exploring sexual identity and preferences. However, it's essential not to overlook the importance of emotional connections and mental well-being in enhancing libido.

The societal pressures and expectations placed upon young adults can significantly impact their sexual desire. Navigating through college, early careers, and newfound independence often brings stress and anxiety, which can dampen libido. It's crucial to recognize that while external responsibilities are unavoidable, creating a balance is key to maintaining a healthy and vibrant sexual life. Prioritizing self-care and stress management can prevent these pressures from overwhelming desire.

Building emotional intimacy is just as vital as the physical aspect when it comes to enhancing libido in young adulthood. At this stage, establishing deep emotional connections can lead to a more fulfilling sexual experience. It's about finding someone who resonates with your values, dreams, and desires. This emotional bond acts as a catalyst for a thriving libido, allowing individuals to express their true selves without fear or reservation.

Communication is the linchpin of any successful relationship, and it is especially critical in this stage of life. Open dialogue about desires, boundaries, and expectations can help partners understand each other better and foster a stronger connection. Understanding one's own needs and being able to articulate them clearly is a practice that can lead to a significantly enhanced and satisfying intimate life.

Additionally, exploring new experiences together can invigorate desire. Engaging in activities that both partners enjoy can stoke the fires of passion. This mutual exploration promotes a sense of adventure and novelty, which are pivotal in keeping desire alive and exciting. It might be as simple as trying a new sport, learning a dance together, or traveling to a new destination—the key lies in sharing experiences and building memories that reinforce the partnership.

Another critical aspect of enhancing libido during young adulthood is body awareness and acceptance. Young adults are often bombarded with media portrayals of 'ideal' bodies, which can skew their perception of beauty and worth. Cultivating a positive body image and self-worth is fundamental to a healthy libido. Recognizing that true sensuality and attractiveness come from within fosters confidence and frees individuals from the constraints of unrealistic standards.

Understanding the mind-body connection is also pivotal during this time. Engaging in regular physical activity not only contributes to overall health but also boosts libido. Exercise releases endorphins, improves mood, and regulates hormones, all of which play a significant role in enhancing sexual desire. Young adults should explore different forms of exercise to find what best suits them, whether it's yoga, running, dancing, or strength training—each offers unique benefits.

Nutrition cannot be overlooked when discussing libido enhancement. A balanced diet rich in essential vitamins and minerals supports hormonal balance and energy levels. Foods such as dark chocolate, nuts, and fruits like strawberries and avocados are known to have aphrodisiac qualities and can be included in meals to naturally boost libido.

Moreover, embracing self-love and self-compassion lays a strong foundation for desire in young adulthood. Acknowledging and honoring personal needs, desires, and boundaries is an act of self-respect that fuels confidence and empowerment. Practices such as mindfulness and meditation can assist in nurturing this self-awareness and acceptance, allowing individuals to stay grounded amidst life's hustle.

In young adulthood, the role of technology also becomes prominent in forming and maintaining relationships. While digital communication tools provide convenience and connectivity, they can sometimes serve as barriers to deep, meaningful interactions. It's important to balance screen time with face-to-face engagements to cultivate genuine connections that fuel intimacy and desire.

Finally, experimenting with sexual techniques and exploring fantasies can lead to an enriched sexual experience. This exploration should be safe and consensual, with communication at its core. Understanding one's likes and dislikes, along with a willingness to experiment within those boundaries, adds a layer of excitement and enhances the overall sexual journey.

Young adulthood is a beautiful, transformative stage of life that offers endless opportunities for growth, learning, and connection. By focusing on emotional intimacy, self-awareness, and open communication, individuals can enhance their libido and cultivate a fulfilling sex life that complements this dynamic phase. Through embracing change and nurturing connections, young adults can navigate the complexities of desire with confidence and joy.

Desire During Parenthood

Parenthood brings a myriad of changes, weaving joy and challenges into daily life, and in the whirlwind, intimate desires can sometimes be placed on the back burner. Yet, maintaining a vibrant libido during this stage is not just possible, it's essential for nurturing a strong partnership. Parenthood, while demanding, can enhance desire by deepening the bond of shared experiences. Couples grow when they embrace the dance between the roles of caregiver and lover, allowing moments of intimacy to blossom within the heart of family life.

Finding time for connection amidst sleep schedules and school runs might seem daunting, but creativity and communication are your greatest allies here. Little gestures of affection, like a lingering touch or spontaneous compliments, go a long way. Recognizing that passion needs tending—much like a delicate seedling requiring water and light—fuels the desire to carve out time for each other. Embracing the fun, mess, and unpredictability of parenthood can actually enrich your romance, creating a love that's rooted in resilience and tenderness.

Managing Parenthood's Impact on one's libido and intimate relationships is a nuanced journey. Parenthood, with all its beautiful chaos and profound joy, can bring unexpected challenges to maintaining desire and intimacy. As life shifts to accommodate new responsibilities, many couples find their romantic lives altered in ways they hadn't anticipated. Instead of letting these shifts become barriers, understanding and adapting to them can pave the way for a deeper, more rewarding connection.

First, it's essential to acknowledge the changes in daily routines that come with parenting. Sleep schedules often become erratic, and attention is divided, leaving little room for spontaneous moments of intimacy. The cumulative fatigue can make even the thought of romance feel overwhelming. To navigate this, it helps to prioritize rest and understand that it's perfectly natural for desires to ebb and flow during this stage. Partners can find solace in the knowledge that they're in this together and that compassionate support is key to transcending these hurdles.

One way to manage parenthood's impact on libido is by consciously carving out time for each other. Consider setting aside regular 'couple's time'—moments that are sacred and just for the two of you, free from the demands of parenting. This doesn't need to be extravagant; even small gestures, like shared coffee breaks or evening walks, can rekindle a sense of closeness. By creating a space to reconnect as partners rather than just parents, you nurture the bond that brought you together in the first place.

Acknowledging the emotional workload can also be transformative. Parenthood often brings an array of emotions, from overwhelming joy to outright frustration. Being open to discussing these feelings candidly with your partner can strengthen your emotional intimacy. Encourage each other to share experiences honestly and without judgment. This space of vulnerability can act as a foundation for boosting the desire that may feel dormant amid parenting chaos.

It's worth exploring the idea of shared activities that are both relaxing and invigorating. Consider engaging in activities that not only restore individual energy but also nourish the relationship. This could include anything from taking up a dance class together, practicing yoga, or engaging in a shared hobby. Activities that build both comfort and excitement help create a versatile space for connection, easing the path back to desire.

For some, the physicality of touch and closeness can reignite the embers of passion that have dimmed. Regular, non-sexual touch— such as holding hands, hugging, or sitting close—fosters a sense of connectedness and warmth. This physical closeness often bridges the gap between everyday partnership and moments of sexual intimacy. It can remind partners of their roles beyond co-parents to lovers, elevating their connections in subtle yet meaningful ways.

Moreover, embracing a mindset of gratitude towards each other can transform your perspective on your partnership amidst parenthood. Reflect on what you appreciate about your partner not only as a co-parent but as an individual. Verbalize these appreciations, making them known. Gratitude can lead to positive emotions and a renewed appreciation that serves as a preliminary step toward a reinvigorated libido.

It's also crucial to manage expectations and redefine what intimacy looks like during this life stage. Understanding that it doesn't have to be extravagant or even frequent can take off the pressure. Relishing in brief moments of connection, whether through a shared laugh or a tender touch, becomes vital. This reconceptualization allows you to redefine intimacy in a way that aligns with your current realities and needs.

Couples might explore avenues outside the norm to keep engagement dynamic—such as writing love notes to each other or planning surprise mini-dates that fit into busy schedules. These gestures remind partners of their dedication to one another and help maintain a palpable romance that parenting responsibilities often obscure.

For some couples, deeper insights might be needed, perhaps in the form of counseling or therapy. Professional guidance can offer tailored strategies to rekindle desire and improve communication, ensuring partners are aligned in their goals and approaches. Seeking help need not be viewed as a sign of failure, but rather a commitment to fostering a thriving and passionate relationship, even amid the demands of parenting.

Finally, don't underestimate the impact of self-care. When individuals take time to care for their mental, physical, and emotional health, they're better equipped to engage meaningfully with their partners. Whether through exercise, meditation, or personal hobbies, investing in oneself is an investment in the relationship's vitality. A well-nourished self naturally attracts a deeper level of connection, enriching both personal and shared experiences of desire.

Managing the double-edged sword of parenthood's demands and its impacts necessitates patience, creativity, and mutual respect. Nurturing intimacy in this stage may take different forms but offers a profound opportunity to cultivate a resilient, adaptive, and loving partnership. As you navigate this journey, embrace the challenges as catalysts for growth and deeper connection, reinforcing the unique bond that parenthood, while transformative, ultimately strengthens.

Tips for Maintaining Passion Parenthood is an extraordinary chapter in life, filled with new discoveries and unparalleled joys. Yet, it brings its own set of challenges, particularly when it comes to maintaining a vibrant intimate connection with your partner. Engaging with your partner during this time requires attention, creativity, and resilience. Passion, like a garden, can bloom beautifully even with the arrival of young ones, provided it's diligently tended to.

Embracing openness in your communication serves as foundational soil for nurturing desire during parenthood. It's essential to share your thoughts, feelings, and needs in a way that reflects not just honesty but compassion. This isn't about perfectly curated conversations but rather creating a safe space for both partners to express where they are mentally and emotionally. Here, empathy plays a role of paramount importance, enabling partners to navigate complex emotions with understanding and support. Appreciating that each other's experiences and stressors are different can foster profound intimacy.

Time management is often the primary hurdle for new parents attempting to sustain their romantic flame. Daily routines are frequently overwhelmed by the seemingly endless demands of newborns or toddlers. Therefore, deliberate scheduling can transform into a powerful ally. While spontaneity has its allure, the disciplined setting aside of 'us time' ensures that your relationship priorities remain clear and honored. Allow yourselves the liberty of crafting this time creatively—short walks, shared chores, or an evening cup of tea could become windows into restoring connection.

Creating ritualistic experiences, even in brief moments, can potentially be a transformative force. Bedtime routines for children, once you find a rhythm, can open up nightly opportunities, however small, for partners to reconnect. Build traditions like 'candlelit conversations' or occasional 'mini home date nights' after the kids have gone to bed. Such rituals bind you together not just in practice but in mind and heart, reinforcing partnership amidst life's busyness.

Remember the power of touch, a cornerstone of connection. Passing hugs in the hall, a warm hand on the back as you pour morning coffee, or a goodnight kiss—these little acts are tokens of affection and reassurance. They are gestures that whisper, "I see you, I remember us." Touch is not only physical but emotional. It's about recognizing the shared journey, all its trials and joys, reaffirming that love extends beyond the immediacy of parenting demands.

Yet, passion—like any emotion—can ebb and flow. Instead of resisting this natural cycle, learning to ride its waves can help keep frustrations at bay. During lulls, lean into understanding, patience, and humor, seeing it as a phase of adaptation. As roles shift and evolve, so too must expressions of intimacy. Playfulness can be a welcome companion, lightening the load that comes with responsibilities and restoring vibrancy in unexpected ways.

In the midst of responsibilities, celebrating small victories together fosters a sense of teamwork and accomplishment. Whether it's the first successful potty-training day or a rare long nap, find delight in these moments. They are occasions to acknowledge the partnership beyond caregiving, honoring the shared commitment that extends deeply into every corner of life.

Parenthood can indeed seem like a maze with unpredictable turns. Yet, nestled in its winding paths exists the potential for deepened love and connection. This journey necessitates embracing the shifts while making intentional choices to nurture the 'us' in your relationship. Every laughter shared, every supporting glance exchanged, adds a vibrant stroke to the painting of your shared life.

In quiet moments, reflect together on the initial spark of your relationship. Recalling the shared dreams, aspirations, and even the wild ambitions from the days before parenthood can serve to reignite those old flickers of desire. Reminiscing isn't about yearning for the past but recognizing the growth journey and hope for the future. This emotional bridge can deepen appreciation for where you've been, where you are, and the dreams you now forge for each other and your family.

Lastly, never underestimate the transformative power of seeking knowledge together. Discuss articles, books, or podcasts focused on relationships or parenting. Jointly exploring new ideas and perspectives can invigorate your dialogue and offer new insights into each other's evolving identities and desires. As you grow—both as individuals and partners—you grant each other the permission to redefine and refresh what passion looks like in this shared chapter.

Maintaining passion through the whirlwind of parenthood is possible. It requires less of grand gestures and more of nurturing every small, intentional interaction. By focusing on communication, time management, touch, adaptability, and shared learning, you can ensure not just the survival, but the flourishing of intimacy and desire in your relationship. Together, you possess the keys to cultivating a love story that deepens and expands with the unimaginably sweet complexity of raising children.

Chapter 16:
Cultural and Societal Influences on Libido

In a world where cultural norms and societal expectations often shape our perceptions of self and relationships, understanding their impact on libido is crucial. Media bombard us with idealized images that can distort our sense of worth and desire, creating unrealistic benchmarks for beauty and passion. Such influences can lead to body image struggles and a diminished sense of self-acceptance, which in turn can suppress libido. However, cultivating media literacy and embracing strategies for self-acceptance can transform these challenges into opportunities for growth. By challenging societal narratives and redefining personal desires within our unique cultural contexts, we can nurture a healthier, more fulfilling sense of intimacy. Embracing diversity, valuing authentic beauty, and fostering open dialogues about cultural norms empower us to strengthen connections and rekindle desire. When we actively engage with our cultural surroundings, rather than resist them, we unlock pathways to a libido that is both resilient and liberating.

Media and Expectations

In today's society, media plays a powerful role in shaping perceptions, especially around concepts of desirability and passion. The barrage of images, movies, and narratives can create a distorted view of what a fulfilling intimate relationship looks like. While some media portrayals can inspire, encouraging an exploration of new perspectives and styles of intimacy, they can also set unrealistic expectations that may hinder genuine connection.

Consider the way romance is depicted in films or advertisements. Often, relationships are depicted as a continuous parade of grand gestures and flawless passion—a depiction that's more fantasy than reality. These portrayals contribute to a cultural script about what desire should look like, often leaving real-life partners feeling inadequate by comparison. When these fictitious depictions shape our expectations, they can lead to feelings of pressure, disappointment, and frustration, manifesting as perceived failures when real-world dynamics don't align.

It's important to recognize the beauty in the ordinary, the genuine in the small and tender moments that aren't typically highlighted on screen. The spontaneous laughter after a shared joke, a lingering gaze that communicates silent understanding, or the soft touch that reassures and grounds us—these are threads woven into the fabric of authentic intimacy. Such moments don't make for cinematic drama but they foster connections that are real, fulfilling, and resilient against the fleeting whims of media trends.

Understanding the influence of media involves acknowledging how it shapes our views on body image and self-worth. The perpetual stream of perfectly edited photos and curated content can set an unattainable standard that fuels insecurity and self-doubt. In doing so, it can dampen an individual's self-esteem and, in turn, their libido. How we perceive and feel about ourselves doesn't exist in isolation; it's deeply connected to how we relate to others. A negative self-image can be a significant barrier to maintaining a healthy and fulfilling sexual desire.

Strategies for cultivating media literacy become essential tools. This includes critical engagement with media content—asking questions about the hidden agendas, recognizing the prevalence of enhancement and manipulation, and proactively seeking diverse representations. Exposure to a broader range of narratives can support growth toward holistic self-acceptance and gratitude for one's unique attributes, counteracting the narrow and often destructive ideals touted in mainstream media.

Let's not overlook the role of social media, a modern powerhouse in influencing personal and societal norms. Platforms designed for connection can breed a form of performance anxiety with users curating a life that fits societal ideals. Social validation through likes and shares becomes a metric for success, shifting focus away from intimate, personal relationships to the depiction of 'desirability' based on external approval. Social networks can build community and offer a space for diverse expressions of identity if navigated with awareness.

To foster healthier expectations and reinforce a genuine connection with oneself and others, we can seek supportive communities and positive online spaces. These environments encourage openness and authenticity, where the exploration of intimacy is celebrated free from judgment or comparison. Building a digital narrative that echoes the values of acceptance and warmth can inspire others to embrace their journey, paving the way for richer, more meaningful interactions both online and offline.

As we examine the interplay between media and expectations, it's clear that the narratives we consume hold significant power. They can mold perceptions, but also provide a platform for redefining what desire means personally and collectively. Empowerment comes from seizing the narrative, interpreting our experiences, and crafting intimate stories that are personal, fulfilling, and genuine.

As partners navigate their paths, finding ways to safeguard the sanctity of their relationship from external pressures becomes essential. This involves not just rejecting unhealthy standards but also embracing conversations about desires and boundaries without judgment. Amidst a world filled with noise, the quiet conversations shared between partners can become powerful acts of resistance and understanding. Here lies the strength to shape expectations not based on media's version of perfection, but on what truly resonates with both partners in the dance of intimacy.

Cultivating a Positive Body Image

In a world inundated with unrealistic standards and pressures from media portrayals, nurturing a positive body image becomes a vital aspect of fostering desire and intimacy. Cultivating self-love and embracing one's unique physique can profoundly enhance an individual's confidence, which is intimately connected to their libido. This journey towards acceptance involves consciously challenging societal norms and embracing diverse representations of beauty. By cultivating a mindset that appreciates the body for its incredible capabilities rather than its perceived shortcomings, individuals can experience a heightened sense of self-worth and desirability. Embracing practices like media literacy helps in filtering out negative influences, while self-acceptance strategies encourage a loving dialogue with oneself. Ultimately, a positive body image not only enhances personal well-being but also deepens the connection with a partner, paving the way for a more fulfilling and intimate relationship.

Media Literacy plays a pivotal role in helping individuals navigate the complex interplay between media messages and personal self-image, all of which impact one's libido. In today's digital age, where media pervades nearly every aspect of our daily lives, it's crucial to understand its influences, particularly in cultivating a positive body image. By empowering ourselves with media literacy, we can develop a more compassionate and realistic view of self-worth that can enhance our intimate relationships and boost desire.

When we talk about media literacy, we're referring to the ability to critically analyze media messages and recognize their underlying intentions. This skill is essential in sorting through the barrage of images and narratives that bombard us from television, magazines, social media, and even advertising. These media forms often present idealized versions of beauty and success that can distort our perception of reality and, consequently, our self-image. With a better grasp of media literacy, you can start to challenge these narratives and form a more authentic understanding of yourself and those around you.

The omnipresent media has a profound effect on our self-perception and, subsequently, on our libido. The portrayal of perfect bodies and flawless relationships can lead to unrealistic expectations that harm self-esteem and intimate connections. By dissecting these portrayals and acknowledging their artificial nature, individuals can break free from these constraints and embrace their unique beauty. Doing so boosts confidence and allows lovers to connect deeply, fostering a healthier sexual relationship.

To cultivate a positive body image, it's crucial to assess the types of media we consume consciously. Consider what types of social media accounts you follow or the shows you watch. Do they support an inclusive representation of bodies and kinds? By choosing media outlets that promote diversity and authenticity, you inadvertently encourage a broader acceptance of different body types. This broader acceptance spills over into your self-perception, positively influencing your libido as you become more comfortable with your own appearance.

Another important aspect of media literacy is understanding the persuasive techniques used by advertisers and content creators. Many media messages capitalize on insecurities, urging consumers to buy products that claim to enhance attractiveness or suggest they need to change certain aspects to be desirable. Recognizing these tactics allows you to sidestep the trap of comparison and inadequacy that can lead to dissatisfaction in your intimate life. Instead, you can focus on nurturing what truly matters: your emotional and physical connection with your partner.

Furthermore, media literacy teaches us to question and decode the content we engage with. Ask yourself why certain images make you feel insecure or why specific narratives seem appealing. Is it societal pressure, or is there a deeper personal story at play? By probing these questions, you become more self-aware and can work towards resolving issues that plague your self-image and dampen your libido.

Consider setting boundaries around media consumption as a step towards media literacy. Limit exposure to content that fosters negative self-talk or imposes unrealistic standards. Instead, surround yourself with positive, affirming messages that celebrate diverse expressions of beauty and intimacy. Engaging with accounts or platforms that promote self-love and acceptance over perfection can be incredibly liberating. As you engage positively with media, it propels a better understanding and acceptance of oneself, uplifting sexual confidence.

This nuanced understanding of media's influence allows for a more grounded perspective and an appreciation of your personal journey. Recognize that everybody's story and expression are unique. By embracing this, you enrich your intimacy with authenticity, thereby boosting your desire and connection. In relationships, authenticity can be a powerful aphrodisiac; when both partners feel accepted and valued for who they truly are, it enhances the emotional and physical dimensions of their bond.

Let's not forget the significance of discussing media's impact with your partner. Have open conversations about how media representations make you feel and share the journey of media literacy together. These discussions can not only fortify your relationship but also create a supportive environment where both feel free to express vulnerabilities. The process of learning together and growing more media savvy can be a bonding experience, solidifying your partnership and rekindling desire.

More practically, media literacy workshops or online courses can offer structured paths to learning. These programs can provide tools and strategies that help individuals navigate the complex media landscape. By such means, the practical application of media literacy turns from a theoretical exercise into a daily practice, reinforcing a positive body image and enhancing your libido.

Incorporating media literacy into your lifestyle isn't just about recognizing and rejecting unrealistic beauty standards; it's about cultivating a sense of empowerment. When you're equipped with the knowledge to question and critique media messages, you become less susceptible to their pressures, fostering a profound sense of agency. This empowerment not only enhances self-image but also enriches intimate relationships, as you become more confident and at peace with who you are.

Media can be a double-edged sword, presenting challenges but also opportunities for growth and connection. Through the lens of media literacy, redefine your relationship with it and, consequently, with yourself. By doing so, you nurture your self-esteem, which directly feeds into a healthy and thriving libido. With an open heart and a critical mind, you can navigate these modern complexities and create a fulfilling intimate life grounded in truth, connection, and love.

Self-Acceptance Strategies Cultivating a positive body image is intricately tied to self-acceptance, a cornerstone for enhancing one's libido amidst cultural and societal influences. In a world teeming with societal pressures and media portrayals of 'ideal' bodies, finding peace with your own can feel like a daunting journey. However, embracing self-acceptance is not only instrumental in fostering a healthy body image but is also a powerful strategy for rejuvenating your intimate life.

Self-acceptance begins with understanding and acknowledging your own uniqueness. The moment you start valuing what makes you uniquely beautiful—be it a feature, a talent, or a unique perspective on life—you lay the groundwork for a positive body image. This understanding can be particularly liberating in countering the ubiquitous, often unattainable, standards set by media. Take a moment to reflect on what you appreciate about yourself, and remember that true attractiveness stems not from conformity, but from authenticity.

Another strategy to cultivate self-acceptance is to practice gratitude. Keeping a gratitude journal where you regularly note down aspects of your body and self that you are thankful for can create a shift in perception. This small but effective practice reminds you to celebrate your capabilities rather than focusing on perceived flaws. Over time, this shift nurtures self-compassion, which is integral to self-acceptance and creating a positive self-image that enhances your sexual desire.

Mindful self-reflection is also key in fostering self-acceptance. Mindfulness can help cultivate a non-judgmental awareness of your body and its sensations. Instead of critiquing your physique, mindfulness encourages you to experience your body as it is in the present moment. Whether it's through mindfulness meditation, yoga, or mindful breathing exercises, such practices encourage a deeper connection with oneself, promoting a harmonious balance between mind and body. This connection becomes especially vital during intimate moments, allowing you to let go of inhibitions and immerse fully in the experience.

Engage in positive self-talk as it plays a crucial role in reshaping perceptions of self-worth and desirability. The narratives we tell ourselves significantly influence our beliefs and actions. Replace self-critical statements with affirmations that highlight your strengths and embrace your individuality. Affirmations like "I am enough" or "I embrace my true self" reinforce positive beliefs, helping to gradually dismantle negative thought patterns imposed by societal expectations.

Connectivity with others who celebrate body diversity can also bolster self-acceptance. Cultivating a supportive community that values and uplifts varied body types offers a sense of belonging and acceptance. Whether through social media groups that promote body positivity or engaging with communities focused on self-improvement and self-love, these connections reiterate that there isn't a one-size-fits-all model for beauty or sexual allure.

Fostering a sense of self-worth is pivotal in this journey. Making a habit of setting and achieving personal goals outside of physical appearance can lead to immense self-satisfaction. By challenging yourself in areas like career, hobbies, or personal projects, you redefine your value spectrum, reducing the emphasis on appearance alone. This expansion of self-worth fosters a self-assuredness that makes you more open to exploring and enjoying intimacy.

Body neutrality is another powerful strategy. Instead of focusing intensively on loving every aspect of your body, which can feel overwhelming at times, you might aim for a perspective where you respect and appreciate your body for what it does for you. Shifting the focus to function over form allows a healthier, more balanced view, paving the way for relaxed confidence both in everyday life and in intimate encounters.

Moreover, redefine your relationship with your body by engaging in activities that make you feel in tune with yourself. This could include dancing, art, or any physical activity that you enjoy which connects you with your body in a joyful way, rather than exercising solely for aesthetic improvements. Such activities can serve as reminders of the pleasure and capabilities your body offers, far beyond meeting visual ideals.

Lastly, it's important to recognize that acceptance itself is a continual process. There might be ebbs and flows in how you feel about your body, and that's perfectly normal. The journey we take with our bodies is ongoing and shaped by numerous factors—emotional, societal, and personal. Accepting this fluidity allows you to be kinder to yourself, reducing pressure and inviting a more genuine and fulfilling approach to intimacy.

Ultimately, adopting self-acceptance strategies within the context of cultivating a positive body image isn't just beneficial—it's transformative. By redefining relationships with our bodies and fostering an atmosphere of self-kindness and compassion, you not only enhance your own libido but glimpse a profound connection with your partner, grounded in authenticity and mutual respect.

Chapter 17:
Planning for Intimacy

In the often hectic pace of our daily lives, carving out moments of genuine intimacy with our partners can become a crucial, albeit overlooked, pursuit. To nurture a connection that thrives, intentional planning can transform intimacy from a spontaneous desire into a cherished ritual. Consider the intimate atmosphere you're cultivating; a dimly lit room with soft music might set the stage for vulnerability and closeness. Scheduling intimate time isn't about reducing passion to an appointment but about prioritizing your relationship amidst life's demands. When you actively create space for intimacy, it becomes a sanctuary where both partners can reconnect, explore desires, and foster deeper bonds. Introducing small rituals, like preparing a favorite meal together or sharing moments of gratitude, further enriches this sacred time. Let these intentional acts of connection be the compass that guides you towards a fulfilled and passionate romantic life.

Creating a Comfortable Environment

Planning for intimacy is an art, a delicate dance that requires the perfect blend of spontaneity and intention. At the heart of this dance is the setting in which intimacy unfolds. **Creating a comfortable environment** is crucial to unlocking deeper connections and sparking passion. It's not just about physical surroundings; it's the emotional and sensory layers that together create an oasis of trust and vulnerability.

Begin by paving the way for comfort with your immediate surroundings. Think about the room where you intend to ignite passion—the lighting, the aromas, the textures. Ambient lighting with soft, warm hues can turn an average space into a haven of romance, soothing the senses while setting a relaxed tone. Candles can invoke a sense of intimacy with their gentle flickers, but be mindful of scents. Some fragrances, like vanilla or sandalwood, gently stimulate without overwhelming the senses.

Arrange the space to eliminate distractions. A cluttered room can lead to a cluttered mind, so take the time to tidy up. Removing unnecessary items is more than aesthetic; it's symbolic. You're choosing to prioritize your partner over the everyday chaos. A carefully curated playlist can sweep unwelcome thoughts away. Music that resonates with both partners creates a shared auditory landscape, a backdrop for the story you're about to write together.

A focus on *physical comfort* can't be overstated. Invest in quality bedding and pillows; soft materials that invite touch and encourage relaxation can make all the difference in the tactile experience. Fabrics that feel good against bare skin enhance sensory pleasure, contributing to overall satisfaction. Adjusting room temperature is a simple yet effective way to ensure comfort. This attention to detail sends a message that nurturing each other's needs is paramount.

Beyond the tangible, creating a comfortable environment involves fostering an atmosphere filled with emotional security. Engage in conversations that reaffirm your connection before delving into intimacy. This includes affirmations of love, shared gratitude, or discussing hopes and dreams. By opening up these channels of communication, partners lay the groundwork for vulnerability and trust. Emotional harmony leads to a cohesive physical bond.

Consider also the power of ritual. Thoughtfully establishing routines before intimacy can signal a transition from the outside world to your shared space. Whether it's sharing a cup of tea or a quiet moment of mindfulness together, these rituals prepare the mind and body, guarding against intrusion from daily stresses. Consistent rituals build a foundation of comfort; you know what to expect and look forward to these moments.

Sometimes, the key to a comfortable environment is simply giving yourselves permission to **let go and be present**. Embrace mindfulness by focusing entirely on the present moment without the burden of expectations or past experiences. It's about being attuned to your partner's needs and responses, creating an intimate feedback loop where touch and communication are in harmony.

Incorporate elements that resonate personally with both partners, fostering a sanctuary uniquely yours. Shared experiences, such as reading a favorite book aloud, or engaging in a simple yet thoughtful activity together, can deepen emotional bonds. Personal touches like framing a meaningful photograph or wearing a cherished piece of jewelry can evoke fond memories and remind you of your journey together.

Don't underestimate the role of humor and playfulness in creating this environment. Laughter relaxes and energizes, breaking down walls and encouraging connection. Playfulness invites creativity and exploration, allowing you to rediscover each other in new ways. Being able to laugh together, particularly during intimate moments, can significantly lower inhibitions and promote a sense of security.

The importance of syncing up mentally and emotionally cannot be overstated. Sometimes, setting aside time for meditation or breathing exercises together can harmonize both your energies, aligning desires and intentions. These practices can create mental space, making room for desire to flourish naturally.

Lastly, appreciate the impermanence and uniqueness of each moment shared. Not every intimate encounter needs to be groundbreaking. Accepting this makes it easier to enjoy the journey rather than focusing solely on a specific outcome. It reminds us that intimacy isn't a destination but a continual process of discovery and connection.

By considering these aspects, you craft an environment where comfort, trust, and passion can thrive. The priority isn't always about reaching a physical pinnacle, but about nurturing a space where both partners feel safe, cherished, and connected. This sets the stage for deeper understanding and shared pleasure, ensuring that intimacy is both a refuge and an adventure.

The Role of Scheduling

In the dance of life's demands, finding time for intimacy can seem like an elusive endeavor, yet its importance cannot be overstated. Scheduling intimate moments might seem counterintuitive to spontaneity, but planning can foster anticipation and commitment to nurturing your relationship. Imagine intimacy not as another responsibility but as a heartfelt commitment to your partner, like setting a date with the person who holds your heart. By intentionally carving out space in your hectic calendar, you create a sanctuary where love and connection are prioritized above all else. It's about crafting meaningful rituals—whether it's a weekly date night or a simple moment to connect each day—that become the cherished threads weaving through the fabric of your relationship. These moments, planned yet filled with genuine emotion, can ignite passion and deepen the bond you share, emboldening your journey toward a fulfilling and intimate partnership.

Making Time for Intimacy is not just about setting aside a few hours for a romantic dinner or a weekend getaway; it's about creating an ongoing commitment to nurture the bond you share with your partner. Amidst the hustle and bustle of daily life, finding moments to connect on a deeper level can seem daunting, yet it is essential for maintaining a fulfilling relationship. The act of scheduling time for intimacy isn't an admission of failure but rather a conscious choice to prioritize what truly matters.

In today's hyper-connected world, distractions are countless. Work emails follow us home, social media beckons at every quiet moment, and the lighting fast pace of life often leaves little room for genuine connection. By deliberately reserving time slots dedicated solely to fostering intimacy, couples can ensure they're continually investing in their relationship. This scheduled time doesn't need to be elaborate or grandiose. Sometimes, the simplest moments can cultivate the deepest connections — a quiet walk, a shared cup of coffee in the early morning light, or embracing silence together as the world rushes by. These small acts, when performed with intention, can wield profound power.

The concept of scheduling intimacy can initially feel mechanical, as if orchestrating love rather than letting it develop naturally. However, consider it as crafting a canvas for spontaneity, rather than prescribing a play-by-play. When the time has been intentionally set aside, you're free to explore whatever arises — whether that's back-to-back episodes of a favorite show, an unexpected culinary adventure, or simply stargazing from your balcony. The anticipation of time spent together can kindle a flame in its own right, turning the mundane into something extraordinary.

Of course, making time for intimacy isn't solely about physical closeness. Emotional intimacy plays an equally critical role. Couples who schedule time for open dialogues often find that their physical connection deepens as well. This may involve sharing personal thoughts, future dreams, or even vulnerabilities. These conversations can reinforce the trust and partnership that underlie a healthy relationship. Emotional intimacy and physical connection feed into one another, creating a cycle of affection and understanding that's integral to a passionate partnership.

For some, the barrier to scheduling intimacy might stem from a fear of routine — that it may dampen the spark that makes a relationship feel alive. But routine isn't the enemy of passion; it can be its greatest ally. Structure provides a safe foundation upon which spontaneity can flourish. Innovative date ideas or surprise gestures can be blended seamlessly with structured plans. For example, you might have a set date night every week, but what you do on that date can vary wildly — from attending a concert to learning a new dance together in your living room.

Creating rituals can be another fruitful avenue within scheduled intimacy. These rituals might be as simple as a regular Sunday morning pancake breakfast or dedicating ten minutes to express gratitude for one another before bedtime. Such rituals anchor the relationship, navigating through life's storms with a sense of togetherness. As these moments become cherished routines, they cultivate an atmosphere of stability and affection.

Another compelling aspect of making time for intimacy through scheduling is the opportunity to align your personal rhythms and discover the times when you are both most receptive to connection. Some partners find morning interactions invigorating, while others discover their best connection late at night. Recognizing and honoring these rhythms can significantly bolster the quality of your intimate moments together.

Navigating life's challenges can often feel overwhelming, where relationships might unintentionally take a backseat. Here, strategy becomes essential. Utilize calendars, reminders, and plans to ensure that you don't drift apart in the face of daily responsibilities. Whether it's marking a calendar with heart symbols or setting weekly alarms labeled "intimacy hour," these acts serve as consistent, gentle nudges toward one another. These reminders not only encourage frequent engagement but send a message that your partnership is prized.

Amidst these strategies, flexibility remains key. There will be days when plans fall through due to unforeseen circumstances. Allow for adaptability, and don't view these as setbacks but as opportunities to revisit and reaffirm each other's importance in your lives. Adjusting plans with grace reinforces that while time together is crucial, understanding and patience are equally so.

While it might seem paradoxical, integrating intimacy into your schedule ensures that it doesn't become just another item on a checklist. It's about creating a tapestry of shared experiences over time that builds up a reservoir of affection and togetherness, ready to draw on in life's trying times. By valuing intimacy enough to schedule it, you reinforce its importance, not just to each other but within the narrative of your shared lives.

Ultimately, making time for intimacy is a declaration — a mutual pledge to embrace life, not in solitary pursuit but as a duo bound by love and shared goals. Whatever form this may take, remember it's not about the clock ticks, but the heartbeats shared within these special moments. In cultivating this practice, you're not just strengthening today's connection but are laying the groundwork for a lifetime of enduring passion and companionship.

Creating Rituals within a relationship offers a sacred space for intimacy, enriching not only the bond between partners but also enhancing the individual sense of connection and desire. A ritual is a shared practice imbued with meaning, something more profound than routine. It transforms the mundane into the magical. These rituals, when intertwined with the daily rhythm of life, can act as anchors, grounding partners in their relationship and creating a sanctuary from the chaos of the outside world. Scheduling these shared intimate moments doesn't strip them of spontaneity; rather, it crafts intentionality that leaves room for organic and heartfelt connections to bloom.

Delving into the art of scheduling intimate rituals requires a mutual understanding and a shared commitment to prioritizing each other amidst life's innumerable demands. It's not about marking a calendar with cold precision but about cultivating moments that become the heartbeat of your relationship. Consider weekly or monthly rituals that both partners can look forward to. It could be as intricate as planning a thematic date night or as simple as making time for a shared sunset walk.

In the modern world, where time is often fragmented and attention spans are stretched thin, creating rituals for intimacy becomes a revolutionary act of love and self-care. It's about being deliberate in a space often left to chance. When partners come together to develop rituals, they engage in a dance of negotiation and creativity. Whether through a cozy Saturday morning in bed with coffee and books or a nightly check-in that culminates in a few minutes of quiet togetherness before sleep, these moments fortify the foundation of a relationship, reinforcing a sense of unity and togetherness.

One compelling way to create rituals is to tailor them around activities both partners find meaningful. It could be a shared interest in cooking, where every week you try a new recipe together, or a mutual love for the arts, perhaps an evening reserved for exploring music or films. The goal is to ensure that these activities don't become mechanical but remain infused with joy and connection. By doing so, partners approach each ritual not with a sense of obligation but with excitement and anticipation.

The first step in creating successful rituals is open communication. Discuss what intimacy means to each of you and how you both wish to experience it. This conversation should be free of judgment and full of vulnerability—a fertile ground for cultivating rituals that feel authentic. As you craft these rituals, remain flexible. What works for one couple may not suit another. Be prepared to experiment and adjust. Rituals, after all, should evolve as your relationship does.

Many couples find that incorporating elements of surprise into their rituals enhances their impact, providing layers of excitement and renewal. Imagine a ritual where one partner plans a surprise element each month. Maybe it's choosing an unvisited spot for a date night or secretly learning a new skill to share with the other. These surprises within rituals can reignite the spark and keep the anticipation alive.

Scheduling to make room for these rituals requires a shared commitment but doesn't demand rigidity. Life throws curveballs, and at times, a scheduled plan may need to navigate life's unpredictability. The key lies in resilience, in the patience to rearrange plans without frustration or disappointment. By maintaining the essence of the ritual—the shared time and intention—even a revised plan can carry the same weight.

Some couples find meditation or shared mindfulness practices to be effective rituals that both enhance intimacy and nurture individual well-being. Starting or ending the day with a brief meditation together can act as a powerful grounding mechanism, directing focus on each other and the present moment. Such rituals don't just connect you with your partner but also align you with yourself, fostering self-awareness and empathy.

Ultimately, creating rituals entwined with scheduling is about fostering a space where desire and intimacy thrive, allowing partners to weave a tapestry of meaningful moments. Remember that intimacy is multidimensional; it's not just about physical closeness but also emotional, intellectual, and spiritual connection. Consider rituals that touch upon these various facets to enrich your relationship fully.

In conclusion, the essence of creating rituals within the framework of scheduling is not to imprison spontaneity but to ensure intimacy can flourish even in the midst of life's hustle and bustle. By dedicating time to rituals and imbuing them with intentionality and creativity, couples can curate a shared life narrative, one rich in connection, love, and mutual growth. Dive deep into this journey with eagerness and a heart open to exploring the boundless possibilities of your shared life map.

Chapter 18:
Exploring Fantasies and Desires

Every relationship carries the potential for an enriching exploration of fantasies and desires, paving the way to deeper connection and understanding. It's about creating a safe, open space where partners can share their innermost yearnings and curiosities without fear of judgment. This gentle dance of vulnerability requires embracing a balance between clear communication of boundaries and the willingness to step into each other's comfort zones. As you examine the landscape of your desires, remember that such exploration isn't a race to a destination but an ongoing journey of discovery. Engage in conversations with curiosity and patience, using these moments to strengthen your bond. Share your fantasies in ways that feel right to you, perhaps by expressing them during pillow talk or jotting them down in a shared journal. Observing each other's responses with empathy can transform how you perceive intimacy, allowing you to weave a tapestry of experiences that resonate uniquely with your shared story.

Safe and Open Exploration

Exploring fantasies and desires in a relationship is an intimate journey, one that requires courage, honesty, and a commitment to openness. It's like unraveling a tapestry woven with threads of passion and curiosity. To embark on this voyage, partners must first create a safe space where vulnerability is welcomed and authenticity is celebrated.

Safe exploration is rooted in both partners feeling secure enough to express their deepest desires without fear of judgment or rejection.

The foundation of safe exploration lies in establishing trust, which acts as the bedrock of intimacy. Trust offers the assurance that your desires, no matter how rare or common, will be met with empathy and understanding. This means being open to listening as much as sharing, creating a balanced dialogue where both voices hold equal weight. When you communicate freely, you're sending a powerful message to your partner: that their desires are seen, heard, and valued.

At the core of this exploration is the concept of consent. It is non-negotiable and should be communicated clearly and respected unfailingly. Consent is what forms the boundary lines within which exploration can safely occur. It's a dynamic conversation that unfolds progressively, adapting as partners grow more comfortable in sharing and experiencing new aspects of their desires. In doing so, you pave the way for genuine connection to foster between you and your partner.

As fantasies begin to surface, the challenge often lies in voicing them. Many grapple with the fear of opening up about desires that might be considered unconventional. Here, understanding and patience play pivotal roles. Partners should encourage each other to share without embarrassment or inhibition. Past experiences, societal taboos, and personal insecurities can cast shadows, but a nurturing environment filled with compassion can illuminate the path forward.

Let's not overlook the power of exploration as a joyful adventure. This should be a time to embrace creativity and playfulness. Introducing elements of novelty and surprise keeps the flame of passion alive, giving couples the freedom to discover aspects of their sensuality previously untapped. Whether it's role-playing, experimenting with scenarios or simply playful discussions, tapping into your inner connoisseur of fun can add vibrancy to the dynamic.

Communicating boundaries is equally essential. It's not just about sharing what you want to explore, but also about conversing regarding what you're uncomfortable with. Healthy exploration thrives on mutual respect and clearly defined limits. Partners should discuss what feels right for them and establish comfort zones where they can retreat if boundaries are approached. Such conversations should be regular, revisiting and reaffirming each other's comfort zones.

Fear of the unknown can sometimes be a barrier to exploration, making the comfort of established patterns appealing. Yet, pushing past that fear is an act of courage that can lead to profound personal growth and an enriched connection with your partner. Be willing to challenge your perceptions and expand the horizons of what intimacy can mean within your relationship. By doing so, you create a sanctuary of love and acceptance where both you and your partner can safely explore your fantasies.

Another aspect of safe exploration is recognizing and honoring each individual's pace. Some may necessitate time to adapt, while others might be eager to dive in headfirst. What's crucial is aligning your rhythms as partners. Stepping to the beat of each other's comfort is a dance of mutual care. Checking in with each other regularly ensures neither feels rushed or bypassed in their process.

Imagine a relationship where both partners confidently unveil their innermost desires without the fear of being misjudged. It's not merely a romantic ideal but an achievable reality when both partners commit to safe and open exploration. This not only enhances your sex life but also strengthens the emotional bond, turning your shared journey into one filled with trust, excitement, and deeper understanding.

So what does it mean to explore safely and openly in practice? Begin by creating a dedicated time and space where conversations about desires can happen naturally and without interruption. It could be as simple as setting aside an evening each week to discuss fantasies or even spontaneous moments where you both feel connected and safe. Remember, the location and timing can significantly impact the quality of your discussions.

Throughout this exploration, keeping curiosity alive is vital. Ask each other questions that invite deeper insight into your partner's desires. Listen with intention and guide the conversation towards mutual discovery rather than focusing solely on individual experiences. Reflect on your shared discoveries and identify new layers of connection that can enrich your partnership. The journey into fantasies should never feel obligatory but should stem from a genuine place of exploration and connection.

In conclusion, exploring fantasies and desires isn't merely about the physical aspects of intimacy but also about delving into the emotional and psychological landscapes of your partnership. Approach each experience with openness and empathy, and you'll find that what starts as a quest to enhance your libido can profoundly elevate the essence of your relationship. This sacred exploration is a testament to the love and dedication you and your partner share, transcending physical desires and transforming intimacy into a heartfelt union.

Communication of Boundaries

The journey of exploring fantasies and desires is exciting, but it demands a strong foundation of trust and open communication about boundaries. Establishing and respecting boundaries creates a safe space where both partners can express their deepest yearnings without fear or judgment. It involves a transparent discussion in which each individual articulates their comfort levels, fears, and limits. This dialogue is not just about setting rules but about nurturing understanding and empathy, ensuring that each partner feels heard and validated in their needs and concerns. As partners share their deepest desires, they should remain attentive to verbal and non-verbal cues that might signal discomfort or hesitation. These conversations, approached with love and patience, empower couples to explore new horizons while maintaining a mutual sense of respect and security. By crafting this supportive environment, couples can transform their fantasies into enriching experiences that deepen their connection and heighten their intimacy.

Establishing Comfort Zones within the dynamic tapestry of exploring fantasies and desires necessitates a nurturing environment where partners feel safe to express their boundaries and curiosities. Communication stands as the cornerstone of this process, providing a platform for honest dialogue and mutual understanding. It's a journey that invites vulnerability, as individuals courageously reveal their deepest desires and establish the limits that keep their exploration enjoyable and secure.

The first step towards establishing comfort zones is fostering an environment where both partners can speak openly without fear of judgment. Authenticity is paramount, as is a willingness to be fully present and to listen. The focus remains on recognizing and respecting each other's comfort levels, as this respect forms the foundation upon which all further exploration is built. Each partner brings unique experiences and expectations that must be acknowledged and valued.

When delving into fantasies, it's vital to remember that they are deeply personal narratives shaped by individual experiences, feelings, and imaginations. As such, allowing each partner the space to express their fantasies without interruption or criticism encourages openness and strengthens trust. The key lies in understanding that revealing these desires is not just an expression of physical longing but is often tied to emotional needs and vulnerabilities.

A nuanced conversation about boundaries goes hand-in-hand with discussing fantasies. It's essential to outline what is acceptable and what isn't within intimate scenarios. This dialogue is not a one-off event but rather an ongoing conversation, a rhythm established between partners that evolves with new experiences and changes in desire. Boundaries can be fluid, needing periodic reassessment as comfort levels shift and grow.

One way to initiate these conversations is by setting aside dedicated time to talk, creating a ritual around these discussions to signify their importance. During this time, partners can explore questions together, such as what each person is curious about, what scenarios might feel daunting, and where each partner's limits currently lie. It's crucial to enter these discussions with compassion, avoiding assumptions about the other's desires and remembering that comfort zones can vary greatly.

Trust plays an indispensable role in these exchanges. When partners know that their boundaries will be respected, they are more likely to venture into new territory without trepidation. Trust allows for a deeper connection and a more honest exploration of desires, encouraging partners to lean into their curiosity while knowing they have the support of their loved one. This mutual trust also enhances intimacy, making each partner feel seen and valued for who they are.

It is helpful to use techniques drawn from exercises in emotional intimacy—such as maintaining eye contact, practicing empathetic listening, and offering affirmations of understanding and support. These techniques are powerful tools in conversations about fantasies and boundaries, giving both partners confidence that they are being heard and understood deeply. Reinforcing these ideas through frequent check-ins can solidify the trust required to explore new dimensions of intimacy.

Another method for establishing comfort zones involves creating non-verbal signals or code words during intimate moments. These can serve as gentle prompts or alerts if a boundary is approaching or has been crossed unintentionally. This system respects each partner's autonomy and ensures an ongoing dialogue even in moments when talking may not be feasible. It stands as a testament to the shared language and trust that partners build together, emphasizing the active, communicative nature of their relationship.

Exploring fantasies does not mean turning every desire into reality. Sometimes, sharing these ideas in the realm of conversation or imagination can be fulfilling in itself. Discussing and even playfully imagining scenarios without the obligation to actualize them can enrich the connection and build a comfort zone where possibilities are endless, but action is always consensual and considered.

Establishing comfort zones is not about eliminating fears or hesitations altogether but about creating a space where these elements can exist alongside excitement and desire. It's about crafting a delicate balance where comfort is maintained without stifling curiosity. This balance requires both partners to be actively involved, to continually refine their understanding of each other, and to celebrate each small step forward in their shared exploration.

Above all, approaching the establishment of comfort zones with patience and a sense of partnership can transform the journey of exploring fantasies from a daunting task into a beautiful, ongoing discovery. Each disclosure, whether of boundary or desire, contributes to a mosaic of intimacy, with each piece reinforcing the shared experience of lovers deeply invested in one another's happiness and fulfillment.

As partners navigate this intricate dance of desires and boundaries, they weave together an intricate landscape of trust and connection. The journey of establishing comfort zones invites them to explore not just their sexual selves, but to embrace each other's totality, learning and growing together in a dynamic, ever-evolving relationship.

Techniques for Sharing Fantasies Sharing fantasies can be a deeply intimate and empowering experience, one that brings partners closer, enhancing both trust and passion. But let's be honest, it can also be a little daunting. The key to this delicate dance lies in understanding not just what fantasies entail but how to communicate them effectively within the realm of boundaries.

First, it's crucial to create a safe space. A safe space isn't just a physical location, but an emotional and mental environment where each partner feels free to express desires without fear of judgment or dismissal. To foster this, begin with an open invitation to talk, ensuring both partners understand that sharing doesn't demand reciprocation, nor does it set expectations. The main goal here is to listen and be heard.

Timing is everything. Choosing the right moment to initiate a conversation about fantasies can significantly impact the outcome. Avoid discussing deep-seated desires when either partner is distracted or stressed. Instead, consider making it part of a relaxing evening together, perhaps over a glass of wine or after a comforting meal. This sets a relaxed tone, dissolving potential barriers to open communication.

Use gentle, exploratory language. Instead of direct demands, try framing your fantasy as a suggestion or curiosity. Phrases like "I've always been curious about..." or "What do you think about trying..." make the conversation a collaborative exploration rather than a one-sided request. This approach can also ease the pressure to fulfill a fantasy immediately, lending the discussion a playful, creative air.

Active listening plays an invaluable role here. Listening isn't just about hearing the words but understanding the emotions and motivations that lie beneath them. Acknowledge your partner's revelations without interrupting and follow up with questions that show genuine interest. Mirroring what you've heard can help solidify trust, for instance, "It sounds like the idea of trying... intrigues you, right?"

Ensure that both partners have equal opportunity to express their fantasies. It shouldn't be a monologue but a dialogue, where each person feels encouraged to partake. Both parties might have different desires that stem from various parts of their identity or past experiences. Recognizing the diversity of fantasies is crucial. They aren't limited to the physical but can also involve emotional or situational scenarios.

It's also essential to discuss boundaries openly. Before diving deeper into certain fantasies, establish what each partner is comfortable with, what might be a hard limit, and what could be a negotiable middle ground. Boundaries aren't static; they're dynamic and can evolve with time and trust. Regular check-ins are vital, ensuring that both partners feel safe and respected as they explore together.

Approach the topic with respect and sensitivity. Remember that fantasies often tap into one's vulnerabilities. Mocking or dismissing them can create a rift rather than promoting closeness. If a particular fantasy doesn't appeal to you, discuss why it might be challenging rather than laughing it off. Empathy and understanding lay the groundwork for deeper intimacy and fulsome conversations.

Create rituals around sharing fantasies to make the process less intimidating and more enjoyable. This could be a monthly 'fantasy night' where each partner anonymously submits desires into a "fantasy jar" to be drawn and discussed. Such rituals infuse predictability and fun into the practice, slowly building comfort and courage in sharing even the bolder fantasies.

Visual aids can also serve as useful tools for communicating fantasies. Using movies, books, or even art can help express ideas that might feel too abstract or embarrassing to articulate. A scene from a film might capture the essence of a fantasy more vividly than words alone could convey, and it offers a concrete reference point for discussion.

Incorporating elements of humor can lighten the atmosphere. While fantasies can be serious expressions of hidden desires, approaching them with a sense of playfulness relieves tension. Laughter and light-heartedness can smooth the way for revelations, reducing the weightiness sometimes associated with such discussions.

Ultimately, sharing fantasies is less about the act itself and more about what it reveals: trust, vulnerability, and a willingness to explore aspects of each other previously undisclosed. The techniques outlined above aim to deepen mutual understanding and connection, acting as a bridge into more authentic companionship and shared intimacy.

Remember that sharing fantasies is an evolving journey. Patience, empathy, and continuous dialogue form the cornerstone of any successful exploration into intimate desires. As partners traverse this path, they may find that their connection becomes not only profound but transformative, fostering a love and intimacy that fulfill beyond imagination.

Chapter 19:
Self-Care and Self-Love

Embracing self-care and self-love is not just a solitary experience; it's a crucial foundation for deepening the intimacy you share with your partner. When you nourish your own wellbeing, you're better equipped to bring vitality into your relationships, rekindling desire and passion. Begin with simple practices of self-compassion, allowing yourself to recognize and honor your needs without judgment. Engaging in mindfulness techniques can keep you present and attuned, enhancing your senses and emotional connections. Develop routines that cherish your individuality—whether it's a quiet walk in nature, a relaxing bath, or a journaling session. As you cultivate love for yourself, you'll find it easier to offer love to others, creating a cycle of nurturing energy and profound connection. This self-awareness not only enhances your personal happiness but also revitalizes the chemistry and intimacy within your partnership, making every shared moment more meaningful and joyous.

Importance of Individual Wellbeing

In the journey toward revitalizing passion and intimacy, the importance of individual wellbeing can't be overstated. Often underestimated, individual wellbeing forms the foundation upon which strong and fulfilling relationships are built. It's a cornerstone that supports not only personal happiness but also the mutual joy and desire shared between partners. When each person in a relationship prioritizes their own wellness, it manifests a ripple effect that enhances connection and intimacy.

Individual wellbeing encompasses both mental and physical health, two aspects that are intricately linked. Caring for your mental health involves nurturing a positive mindset, developing resilience, and acknowledging emotions without judgment. This self-awareness leads to a more profound understanding of your own desires, wants, and needs, which is crucial when fostering a satisfying intimate relationship. It means actively engaging in practices that promote peace and fulfillment, like mindfulness meditation or engaging in creative activities that bring joy.

Physical wellbeing, on the other hand, focuses on maintaining a healthy body through exercise, nutrition, and adequate rest. Regular physical activity releases endorphins, those feel-good hormones that naturally boost mood and increase libido. Eating a balanced diet not only fuels your body but also influences your sexual health and desire. It's about creating a harmonious balance in your physical state that supports an energetic and enthusiastic approach to intimacy.

Moreover, setting aside time for personal interests and self-care routines is just as vital. Engaging in hobbies or pursuing passions can invigorate the spirit, reducing stress and ultimately leaving more energy for partners and shared activities. When one feels fulfilled individually, they bring that sense of accomplishment and positivity into their relationship, creating a nurturing environment for love to thrive.

It's essential to recognize that self-care is not a luxury, but a necessity. In a world that often glorifies busyness, taking time to recharge should be seen as an investment in your relationship. When both partners make self-care a priority, it minimizes burnout and allows for more patience and empathy within the relationship. It becomes evident that when individuals feel contented and cherished by themselves, they are more likely to express love and appreciation outwardly.

Translating this concept into everyday practice involves being intentional with your time and boundaries. It could mean taking a walk in nature, enjoying a quiet cup of coffee in the morning, or writing in a journal to process thoughts. These seemingly small acts create a buffer against the daily stress that can dampen desire and energy levels. When you take care of yourself, you signal to your partner the importance of self-love, promoting a shared value system that encourages both individual and mutual happiness.

Moreover, committing to personal wellbeing means understanding and respecting each person's space and individuality. It's about acknowledging that while you are a unit, you are also unique individuals with separate identities and needs. This respect aids in maintaining a healthy balance between togetherness and independence, a dance that strengthens your bond and enriches your shared life experiences. It allows you to bring your most authentic self to the relationship, cultivating a deep, unshakeable connection.

Finally, let's not forget the spiritual aspect of wellbeing—whatever that may mean for you. Whether it is exploring a belief system, practicing gratitude, or finding solace in quiet reflection, spiritual wellness speaks to the core of many people's sense of being. It provides grounding, perspective, and a bigger picture mindset, which can be incredibly supportive when weathering the inevitable ups and downs of a relationship. Engaging with this facet can nurture an internal peace that radiates outward, inviting a harmonious relationship built on love and understanding.

Ultimately, embracing individual wellbeing is about cherishing yourself as you are, accepting imperfections, and celebrating personal growth. This self-acceptance creates a solid base upon which the intricate dance of a relationship can flourish, nurturing a vibrant and fulfilling intimate life. So, take the plunge into self-discovery and self-care—it's one of the most loving acts you can do not just for yourself but for your partner as well. By fostering your own wellbeing, you nurture the garden of intimacy, where passion and connection can bloom freely.

Practices for Self-Compassion

Practices for self-compassion invite you to embrace your imperfections, fostering an environment where honest affection and understanding flourish not only within yourself but also in your intimate relationships. By acknowledging your worth and practicing self-kindness, you create a ripple effect that enhances your connection with your partner, weaving warmth and emotional depth into your shared experiences. Engage in small acts of mindfulness, like taking a few moments each day to reflect on what you appreciate about yourself, allowing this gentle self-awareness to enhance your desire and intimacy. Cultivating compassion towards your own journey elevates the emotional intimacy you share, nourishing the foundation of desire and paving the way for an enriching and harmonious love life.

Mindfulness Techniques provide a pivotal pathway towards deepening self-compassion, a cornerstone for nurturing self-care and enhancing intimate connections. In the realm of self-love, mindfulness isn't just about cultivating awareness; it's a powerful tool to unlock a more profound understanding of yourself and your desires. At its essence, mindfulness offers a gentle invitation to be present with yourself without judgment, which can transform the way you perceive your needs and emotions—essential elements for a fulfilling intimate life.

Engaging in mindfulness isn't about achieving an enlightened state but rather about embracing the current moment with awareness and acceptance. Imagine sitting in a quiet space, closing your eyes, and focusing on your breath. This simple act of drawing attention to your breathing creates a bridge from the hustle of everyday life back to a more serene state of being. It helps in anchoring your thoughts and feelings, allowing you to gradually release anxieties that might cloud your self-perception and hinder your desires.

Spontaneity often plays a crucial role in romantic relationships, but it's the mindful practice of truly being in the moment with your partner that can elevate these experiences. Imagine sharing a prolonged gaze, where the world fades, and all that exists is a profound connection between you and your loved one. Such moments don't happen by accident; they are cultivated through mindfulness. As you grow more attuned to your inner world, you may find an enhanced capacity to connect deeply with the person with whom you share your life.

Incorporating mindfulness into your daily routine doesn't require significant blocks of time. Even setting aside five minutes each day to focus inward can yield significant benefits over time. It's about forming a habit that shifts your baseline state towards tranquility and presence. Start with a mindful walk or by observing your surroundings with an intentional focus. These practices could be game-changers, leading to an improved sense of well-being and increased libido, as a calm, centered mind opens up new avenues for desire.

While some might perceive self-love as an indulgence, it's actually a necessity—a foundational element that quietly nurtures every aspect of libido and intimacy. In practicing mindfulness, you're giving yourself permission to experience the fullness of who you are, without the criticisms or limitations often imposed by external influences. This form of compassionate self-awareness allows you to better understand your impulses and desires, aligning them with a genuinely loving approach toward yourself.

Consider integrating guided mindfulness practices into your routine. There are numerous online resources and apps designed to gently guide you through meditation and mindfulness exercises. Find a voice that resonates with you, allowing their guidance to lead you into a deeper state of relaxation and self-exploration. It's about finding what works for you and embracing it as part of your daily ritual in a way that enhances the love you hold for yourself and your partner.

One particular technique that marries mindfulness and self-compassion effectively is loving-kindness meditation (LKM). This practice involves silently repeating phrases that invoke feelings of goodwill and love towards yourself and others. As you cultivate compassion within yourself, it naturally extends outward to those around you, fostering a more harmonious relational environment. Such a practice can be transformative, not just in relationships but in your overall approach to life.

Moreover, mindfulness involves a level of courage—to be still, to listen to what arises, and to allow yourself to be without immediate reaction. When you apply this mindset to understanding your libido, you can begin to unravel patterns or beliefs that might have been suppressing your natural urges. It's about nurturing a dialogue with yourself, where curiosity replaces criticism and acceptance trumps judgment.

The pathways to nurturing a rich and vibrant libido through mindfulness and self-compassion are as varied and unique as the individuals who embark upon them. Some may find solace and enrichment in a daily meditation practice, while others might weave mindful moments throughout their day—for example, taking a mindful pause before meals or during routine activities. The key is to turn these moments into opportunities to reconnect with the essence of who you are.

As we focus on developing practices for self-compassion within the context of self-care, the importance of consistency cannot be overstated. Building a regular practice takes determination and a willingness to prioritize yourself, but the rewards—a more profound connection with your desires and an enhanced capacity for intimacy—are more than worth the effort. Remember, this journey isn't about arriving at a perfect state; it's about allowing yourself the space and grace to explore your boundaries and embrace your vulnerabilities.

In conclusion, engaging with mindfulness techniques can ignite a deeper level of self-compassion, serving as a catalyst for not only personal growth but for the richness of your intimate life. As you embrace these practices, you may find that not only does your sense of self flourish, but your connection with your partner blossoms as well. It's through this understanding and compassion that we truly begin to live, love, and desire with intention and authenticity, fostering an environment where passion and intimacy thrive unabated.

Self-Care Routines are the framework of practical habits that emphasize nurturing oneself, both physically and emotionally. These routines are not just pleasant diversions; they play a critical role in enhancing one's capacity for self-compassion, directly influencing how desire and intimacy are experienced and expressed in relationships. Adopting effective self-care routines can pave the way for rekindling desire by first connecting with ourselves, allowing us to engage more authentically and deeply with our partners.

Self-care starts with understanding your body's needs and respecting its signals. This can mean listening to your need for rest, nourishing it with the right foods, or moving it in a way that keeps you energized and grounded. Whether through a rejuvenating morning jog or a quiet evening yoga session, physical activities form the basis of a self-care routine, releasing endorphins that elevate mood and relieve stress. With a clearer mind, partners can be more present with each other, enhancing emotional and physical intimacy.

Incorporating mindfulness into your day serves as another cornerstone of self-care. Small practices like meditation or deliberate deep-breathing sessions help center our thoughts, increasing our awareness of the present moment. This heightened state of awareness makes it easier to appreciate the subtleties of life with a partner, creating an environment ripe for intimacy. By being more attuned to our thoughts and emotions, we foster a deeper connection with ourselves, which naturally extends to those we love.

Emotional self-care is equally important and often begins with the simple act of acknowledging one's feelings without judgment. Taking the time to journal, practice gratitude, or engage in therapy can provide clarity and healing. This process of self-reflection and emotional release clears the way for compassion towards oneself, allowing for greater patience and empathy in interactions with others. When equipped with emotional resilience, couples can navigate the complexities of intimacy with greater ease and understanding.

For couples, self-care doesn't always have to be a solitary pursuit; indeed, shared routines can strengthen bonds. Cooking a healthy meal together, spending a quiet evening unwinding with shared hobbies, or embarking on a mindfulness retreat can deepen understanding and affection. These shared experiences foster a sense of partnership and collaboration, crucial elements in a thriving intimate relationship.

Sleep hygiene is another essential aspect of self-care that boosts libido and helps maintain a sound state of mind. Prioritizing sleep can be remarkably transformative, as adequate rest is intrinsically linked to hormonal balance and stress management. A well-rested individual is often more energetic and emotionally equipped to engage with their partner, both intimately and emotionally. Simple habits such as maintaining a consistent sleep schedule and creating a restful bedroom environment can yield significant benefits.

Lastly, carving out personal time for self-expression is invaluable. Whether it's through art, music, or any creative endeavor, self-expression allows individuals to explore and release inner thoughts and desires. Encouraging a partner to do the same fosters mutual respect for each person's individuality, enhancing the partnership's depth. When both partners embrace their own passions, they bring a more vibrant, fulfilled version of themselves to the relationship, enriching the shared journey.

In nurturing these self-care routines, we lay a foundation for increased resilience, vitality, and affection in our relationships. These practices empower individuals, creating a shared space of enhanced intimacy and mutual respect. With each partner contributing to this space with openness and self-awareness, desire is naturally rekindled, leading to a more passionate and fulfilling connection.

Chapter 20:
Holistic Approaches to
Improving Libido

A harmonious blend of mind, body, and spirit paves the way for deeply enriching intimate connections, and holistic approaches provide a comprehensive path to revitalizing libido. Tapping into the symbiotic relationship between mental well-being and physical health, techniques like yoga and meditation foster a balanced life force, while practices such as acupuncture and reflexology align the body's natural energies. This integration acknowledges that our desire thrives not just in isolation but within the context of our overall lifestyle and health journey. By embracing these ancient and modern integrative therapies, couples can unlock a more profound understanding and appreciation of their desires, creating a sanctuary where passion can flourish naturally. This chapter invites you to explore how nurturing your entire being sets the stage for a vibrant and fulfilling love life, reminding us that true connection is a dance between the physical and the soulful.

Mind-Body Connection

In the dance of desire, the mind and body are not separate partners but intertwined, influencing each step with a fluid grace that cannot be ignored. Our bodies respond to our thoughts and emotions, while our minds, in turn, are influenced by our physical state. Understanding this intricate interplay is key to unlocking the full potential of our libido. When we begin to appreciate the symbiotic relationship between mind and body, we open doors to deeper intimacy and heightened bliss.

Imagine the mind as a conductor, directing an orchestra where the body performs an intricate symphony of sensations. When stress and anxiety cloud the conductor's vision, the music falters, and desire wanes. That's why managing the mind's influence can profoundly impact sexual desire. Techniques like mindfulness and meditation act as gentle reminders for the mind to stay present, enabling us to connect more intimately with our partners.

The mind-body connection can be seen in how our thoughts directly alter physiological responses. Take, for example, how stress triggers the release of cortisol, a hormone that can dampen libido. Alternatively, positive thinking and mental relaxation encourage the production of endorphins, the body's natural mood boosters that enhance arousal. By fostering a positive mental environment, we can cultivate the optimal conditions for desire.

Emotional wellbeing plays a crucial role in this connection. When we're emotionally balanced, we're more receptive to intimacy. Practices that promote happiness and reduce negative inner dialogue—like gratitude journaling or self-affirmations—can empower both mind and body, revitalizing our sexual energy. It's essential to recognize that mental health deserves the same attention as physical health when seeking to enrich one's love life.

One particularly captivating aspect of the mind-body relationship is the placebo effect; the belief in the power of something can sometimes create tangible effects. This underscores the incredible power our minds wield over our physical selves. Harnessing this power involves cultivating a mental landscape that actively supports sexual vitality. Visualization exercises, where one imagines a desired outcome, can change perceptions and even realities, leading to an enriched sensual experience.

While many might dismiss the spiritual aspect of the mind-body connection, spiritual practices can deeply enhance one's awareness and attunement to bodily sensations. Yoga, a practice that marries the physical with the mental through breath and movement, can invigorate one's sense of self and presence. As an integrative approach, yoga offers a pathway to embody balance and harmony, revitalizing both the physical and emotional facets of desire.

Furthermore, the role of sleep in maintaining the mind-body connection should not be underestimated. Restful sleep rejuvenates both mental acuity and physical stamina, vital for sustaining libido. Sleep champions our recovery processes, allowing hormone levels to stabilize and mental burdens to lighten. Prioritizing good sleep hygiene, therefore, is a compelling investment in one's sexual health.

In essence, a nourished mind naturally leads to a flourishing body. Engaging in consistent mental practices like meditation, fostering emotional connections through open dialogue, and being physically active harmonize the mind-body relationship. Each approach represents a step toward understanding—not just fleeting sexual satisfaction—but sustained, joyful desire.

As you embark on this journey of exploration and growth, remember that nurturing the mind-body connection can lead to not just improved libido but a more fulfilling, harmonious life. Enriching this connection with patience and intention can unfold new dimensions in your intimate relationships, deepening bonds in ways you might never have imagined.

Integrative Therapies

Integrative therapies serve as a profound bridge between the mind and body, fostering a holistic approach to enhancing libido. These practices, such as yoga and meditation, encourage mindfulness and relaxation, helping to align physical sensations with emotional experiences. Through the gentle flow of yoga, individuals can improve flexibility and circulation, essential factors for physical intimacy, while meditation aids in reducing stress and fostering emotional connection. Acupuncture and reflexology not only revive physical vitality but also unlock and harmonize energy pathways, often leading to an increase in desire and intimate pleasure. By weaving these therapies into daily life, individuals may find that they deepen their connection with themselves and their partners, creating a robust foundation for passion and intimacy. Integrative therapies invite you to embark on a journey where traditional practices meet modern understanding, offering pathways to fulfill an enriched and connected love life.

Yoga and Meditation are two intertwined practices that provide a profound pathway for enhancing both physical and emotional aspects of libido. Within the broad spectrum of holistic approaches, yoga and meditation stand out as transformative choices that not only connect mind and body but also cultivate a deeper awareness and appreciation of one's self and one's partner. They offer a gentle yet powerful means of peeling away layers of stress and tension, often considered primary roadblocks in desire and intimacy.

Embarking on the journey of yoga invites individuals and couples alike to explore the strengths and vulnerabilities of their own bodies—both independently and in relation to one another. As practitioners flow through poses, they're encouraged to tune into their own physical sensations. This heightened physical awareness extends beyond the yoga mat, fostering better physical connections with partners. Whether it's through a series of sun salutations or more grounding poses geared towards relaxation, yoga helps individuals release pent-up tension that may otherwise impede sexual desire.

Meditation, on the other hand, serves as a vessel for mindfulness—a state of being fully present and conscious in the moment. This practice is invaluable when seeking to enhance libido; being mentally present during intimate moments deepens the connection between partners, improving the quality of their interactions. Through meditation, one learns to quiet the incessant chatter of the mind, allowing for a more profound emotional and sensual presence. It encourages patience and openness, creating space for genuine emotional and physical intimacy.

A unique benefit of yoga and meditation in the realm of intimate connections is their ability to harmonize the body's energy systems. By tapping into ancient traditions such as the chakra system, practitioners gain insights into energies that may be blocked or imbalanced, contributing to diminished libido. Specific yoga poses and meditative practices aim to balance these energy centers, particularly those associated with personal power and sensuality, which can lead to a reinvigorated sense of desire.

For couples who practice yoga and meditation together, these activities become powerful shared experiences that nurture trust and vulnerability. Partner yoga poses, requiring a blend of balance and communication, demand teamwork and understanding. As couples assist and support one another through movements, they learn to rely on mutual cooperation and communication, fostering a deeper bond that translates into their intimate lives.

Consider integrating breathwork, a component common to both yoga and meditation, as part of a daily practice. Breathwork techniques, such as ujjayi or the alternate nostril breath, promote relaxation and arousal by increasing oxygen flow through the body and calming the nervous system. As partners practice controlling and synchronizing their breaths, they forge a sensual rhythm and connection that's both soothing and stimulating.

Cultivating a regular practice of yoga and meditation can also lead to significant stress reduction, helping to counteract one of the most common libido inhibitors. By establishing a routine practice, individuals create a personal space for grounding and self-reflection. For many, this newfound tranquility helps to replace stress-induced adrenaline with serotonin and oxytocin, hormones associated with pleasure and bonding.

Moreover, yoga and meditation offer a non-judgmental environment where individuals can explore and accept their bodies. This acceptance is pivotal when considering body image's impact on sexual desire. Yoga encourages practitioners to embrace their physical selves by fostering self-love and body appreciation, often leading to an enhanced confidence that spills into intimate encounters, making them richer and more fulfilling.

Ultimately, the synergy of yoga and meditation creates an integrative approach capable of catapulting desire and enhancing intimacy. Their profound ability to connect mental with physical, self with partner, offers a potent and lasting pathway to a more vibrant and fulfilling love life. In embracing these practices as part of an integrative therapy, individuals and couples align themselves with a holistic outlook on sexual wellbeing—one that honors and harmonizes the body, mind, and spirit.

Acupuncture and Reflexology are ancient practices that have found a place in modern integrative therapies for enhancing libido, offering powerful, holistic approaches to rekindling desire. Both techniques focus on the body's natural energy flow and pressure points, aiming to restore balance and promote overall wellness. By understanding the benefits of these methods, couples can explore new pathways to intimacy and deepen their connections.

Acupuncture, a cornerstone of traditional Chinese medicine, utilizes fine needles inserted at specific points on the body to stimulate energy flow, or "qi". For many, it's not just about the physical process but the opportunity to engage deeply with one's body in a mindful way. It's believed that acupuncture can potentiate the release of endorphins, alleviate stress, and improve circulation, all of which are crucial in boosting libido. Scientific studies suggest that acupuncture may help address sexual dysfunction, making it a valuable technique for those seeking alternative remedies when conventional treatments fall short.

Reflexology operates on a similar principle but focuses on applying pressure to particular areas of the feet, hands, and ears that correspond to different body systems. This practice is rooted in the idea that these points are linked via a network of pathways, similar to the ones emphasized in acupuncture. Reflexology can enhance relaxation, reduce anxiety, and improve overall bodily function, promoting a conducive environment for intimate connections. By alleviating tension and facilitating the body's natural ability to heal and balance itself, reflexology often leads to improved sexual vitality.

One compelling aspect of these practices is their accessibility; they don't require extensive resources or specialized knowledge beyond finding a trained practitioner. This ease of access makes acupuncture and reflexology attractive options for individuals and couples looking to enhance their libido naturally. As part of an integrative approach, these methods can complement lifestyle changes, nutritional adjustments, and other holistic practices to create a comprehensive plan for improving intimacy.

Couples may find the shared experience of participating in these therapies an additional bond-strengthening activity. Attending sessions together can foster a sense of shared commitment to improving their relationship and sexual health. The trust and communication built through experiences like these are invaluable, nurturing both emotional and physical intimacy.

It's essential to approach these therapies with an open mind and a willingness to explore their benefits over time. Immediate results aren't always guaranteed, but consistent, mindful participation can yield significant improvements in overall wellbeing and sexual drive. Of course, anyone considering these treatments should consult with healthcare professionals to ensure they're appropriate for their particular needs and conditions.

By weaving acupuncture and reflexology into a regular self-care regimen, individuals can harness the transformative power of these practices to revive traditional concepts of intimacy and renew passion in their relationships. This integrative path not only focuses on the physical aspects but incorporates emotional and spiritual dimensions, offering a truly holistic approach to enhancing libido.

As we venture further into this realm of holistic therapies, it's evident that such practices hold the potential to reshape how we understand and cultivate intimate connections. By merging science with ancient wisdom, acupuncture and reflexology continue to serve as guiding lights in the pursuit of fulfilling lovemaking, offering a renewed sense of passion and depth in romantic relationships.

Chapter 21:
Understanding Sexuality and Gender Differences

Embracing the complexities of sexuality and gender doesn't just provide insight; it enriches the intimate connection between partners, paving the way for a more fulfilling romantic life. In today's diverse world, understanding the nuances of sexual orientation and gender identity becomes paramount to fostering love and respect within relationships. By recognizing and valuing these differences, we're not only respecting individual identities but also deepening the emotional and physical bonds that define our personal connections. It's vital to approach these conversations with openness and a willingness to learn, allowing partners to explore desires and identities without judgment or fear. Celebrating and integrating inclusive approaches into our relationships can transform the way we experience passion and intimacy, ensuring that every moment spent together is filled with genuine acceptance and love.

Sexual Orientation and Libido

Understanding the intricate tapestry of sexual orientation and libido is vital to enhancing one's intimate connection and reigniting the flames of desire. Sexual orientation—whether heterosexual, homosexual, bisexual, or any other orientation—plays a profound role in shaping an individual's libido and their approach to sexuality. By embracing the unique qualities of one's orientation, individuals and couples alike can foster a deeper intimacy that is enriched by authenticity and mutual respect.

Sexual orientation is not just about whom one is attracted to; it encompasses one's entire sexual identity and how they perceive and connect with others. This understanding of self is pivotal in shaping a healthy libido. When individuals dare to explore their true orientation, without societal restraints or personal fears, their libido often responds with a natural, uninhibited curiosity and resilience. This sense of liberation and authenticity is critical in forging meaningful bonds with partners, where both desire and passion can flourish without bounds.

Furthermore, acknowledging and embracing one's sexual orientation can contribute enormously to emotional wellbeing, which is directly correlated with sexual desire. When a person feels confident and at ease with their sexual identity, it's likely to manifest in their libido as a spontaneous and fervent expression of affection and intimacy. Emotional stressors, such as the fear of societal judgment or self-doubt regarding one's orientation, can significantly dampen libido, underscoring why acceptance and self-love are crucial.

Libido, the intrinsic drive towards sexual activity, is influenced not only by orientation but also by an array of psychological and physiological factors. It's important to note that the expression of libido can differ drastically across the spectrum of sexual orientations. For instance, studies suggest that cultural and societal norms related to a person's orientation can either constrain or liberate their sexual desires, highlighting the complex interplay between environment and individual sexual drive.

In relationships where partners hold differing orientations or nuances within the same orientation, open and empathetic communication becomes the cornerstone for sustaining and enhancing libido. When partners are candid about their desires, preferences, and boundaries, they craft a shared space where expectations align with realities, creating fertile ground for libido to thrive. Genuine conversations about orientation and sexual desires help in dismantling misconceptions and building trust, thereby boosting the overall passion in the relationship.

Moreover, exploring and understanding the nuances of sexual orientation can spark a renewed interest in sexual exploration for couples. Diverse orientations bring with them myriad perspectives on intimacy and sexual expression, each contributing uniquely to the kaleidoscope of human desire. Couples can continually innovate their intimate practices by integrating these perspectives, nurturing a dynamic sexual relationship that evolves and adapts over time.

Developing a robust libido within any orientation requires sensitivity to one's mental and physical health. Mental health support, for instance, is invaluable in addressing internal conflicts related to sexual orientation that can influence desire. Seeking therapy and counseling can offer individuals and couples essential insights and strategies to embrace their orientations wholly, leading to a liberated and lively libido.

Ultimately, a fulfilling sexual life is one celebrated in tandem with one's sexual orientation. By understanding and respecting individual differences in orientation and how they affect libido, individuals and partners can craft intimate connections rich with understanding, fervor, and mutual joy. This journey of exploration and acceptance is indeed one of the most rewarding paths towards a vibrant and ecstatic intimate life, filled with empathy, connection, and boundless love.

Gender Identity and Desire

Understanding the intricate dance between gender identity and desire is essential for deepening the intimacy within relationships. Gender identity influences how individuals perceive themselves, their roles in relationships, and ultimately how they experience desire. It is a personal journey, often interwoven with societal expectations and personal introspections. Recognizing and respecting these unique identities can unlock deeper levels of passion, encouraging partners to embrace authenticity without fear or judgment. It's about fostering an environment where each person feels valued and seen for who they truly are, creating a space where desire can flourish unhindered by stereotypes. By nurturing open and affirming dialogues, partners can connect more profoundly, aligning their experiences and desires in a harmonious symphony of love and acceptance.

Inclusive Approaches in understanding the nuanced relationship between gender identity and desire are not just beneficial, but vital for fostering deeper, more meaningful connections. As we explore the intersection where sexuality and individuality meet, it is imperative to create spaces where everyone feels seen, heard, and valued. Only by embracing diversity can we truly enhance intimacy and desire within relationships. Let's dive into how inclusivity can transform the narrative around gender identity and desire.

Understanding gender identity requires a shift away from binary thinking. Society has traditionally viewed gender as a strict male-or-female construct. More inclusive approaches acknowledge the spectrum of gender identities beyond this binary, including non-binary, genderqueer, and genderfluid identities. By recognizing this spectrum, individuals and couples can open the door to authenticity and vulnerability, crucial ingredients for intimacy.

Diverse gender identities bring with them varied experiences of desire and attraction. Recognizing and respecting these differences cultivates a sense of partnership and belonging. When discussions about desire are grounded in acceptance, they encourage open, honest communication. This in turn empowers couples to express their true selves without fear of judgment, paving the way for enhanced connection and a more fulfilling intimate life.

Within the space of a relationship, it's essential to explore and honor each partner's unique narrative. This includes understanding how gender identity might influence one's experience of desire. For instance, some trans individuals may find that their sense of desire shifts with hormone therapy or other gender-affirming processes, while others might not. The goal is to cultivate a supportive environment where all experiences are valid and valued.

An inclusive approach also demands that we examine the stereotypes tied to gender roles and desire. These societal norms often dictate who is "supposed" to want what, leading to misunderstandings and frustrations in relationships. By challenging these preconceptions, partners can make room for individualized expressions of desire that reflect true wants and needs rather than societal expectations.

Incorporating inclusive practices in intimate relationships is not merely about providing a theoretical understanding of gender or sexuality. It's about cultivating empathy and providing practical support. For example, regularly checking in with your partner on how they feel about their gender or sexuality can build trust. Open-ended questions, active listening, and empathy all play an essential role in validating their experience.

An active move towards inclusivity in desire also involves acknowledging your own biases and educating yourself. This might mean seeking out diverse media narratives or discussing experiences with others who have different perspectives on gender and desire. Such actions demonstrate a commitment to growth and understanding, fostering a more inclusive environment within your relationship.

Moreover, inclusive approaches should also involve creating a safe space for discussing personal boundaries and preferences. Partners should feel empowered to communicate desires and limits without the fear of rejection or invalidation. Understanding that desires are complex and multifaceted can help partners engage with each other in more meaningful and considerate ways.

Consider setting aside time for conversations specifically focused on exploring and understanding these layers of identity and desire. This can be through reflective dialogue, joint readings, or attending workshops together. The aim is to deepen relational understanding and celebrate the beauty of diversity in identity and desire.

Beyond individual relationships, creating inclusive communities and platforms where diverse narratives of gender and desire are shared can enrich everyone's understanding. Online spaces, support groups, and educational workshops that focus on inclusivity can be invaluable resources, offering support and guidance for both individuals and couples on their journey to embracing diversity.

Let's remember that inclusion isn't a static achievement but an ongoing journey. It requires an open mind, a willingness to learn, and a commitment to empathy. By prioritizing inclusivity in matters of gender identity and desire, we not only enhance personal connections but contribute to a broader culture of acceptance and understanding. This shift can lead to richer, more connected relationships, characterized by genuine desire and lasting intimacy. Inclusivity transforms not just how we love but how we live, in all its beautiful complexity.

Respecting Individual Differences in the context of gender identity and desire means acknowledging and embracing the myriad ways people experience and express their innermost selves. At its core, it's a commitment to understanding and honoring the unique characteristics that make each person who they are. This respect isn't just about acceptance; it's an active choice to celebrate diversity and create space for all identities to thrive, particularly when it comes to intimacy and the nuances of desire.

In today's world, the spectrum of gender identity is as vast as it is intricate, with countless possibilities that go beyond the binary understanding of male and female. This complexity serves as a beautiful reminder that human experience isn't one-size-fits-all. Recognizing this spectrum can enrich intimacy between partners by encouraging a more profound exploration of what each person truly yearns for and values in themselves and their relationships.

Imagine a world where everyone feels seen and heard in their unique gender identity. In relationships, this would foster an environment of genuine openness and empathy. Partners who engage in this practice can communicate more deeply, sharing not only the labels they may or may not associate with but also the emotions and desires that accompany these identities. Such communication nurtures a bond more authentic and meaningful than conventional labels might suggest.

This respect for individual differences in gender identity is not only transformative for partnerships but is essential for personal growth. When individuals are free to explore and express their gender identity without fear of judgment or recrimination, they often experience a liberation that permeates their whole being. This sense of freedom can reignite desire, both individually and within the relationship. Partners, freed from the constraints of societal expectations, can find new ways to connect and engage with one another.

It's crucial to dispel myths and misconceptions that might overshadow our understanding of gender identity and desire. Many mistakenly believe that acknowledging a broad spectrum of gender identities complicates intimacy. In reality, respecting these differences can deepen connection, allowing partners to understand and appreciate each other's unique desires. By setting aside preconceived notions and approaching each other with curiosity and respect, partners can unlock new levels of intimacy and passion.

However, respecting individual differences requires commitment and continuous effort. It involves actively listening to your partner, asking questions, and being willing to uncover the layers of identity that shape each person's experience. This process can be incredibly rewarding, creating opportunities for deeper understanding and more fulfilling intimacy. Furthermore, this effort is a testament to the love and respect partners hold for each other, reinforcing the foundations of their relationship.

For those seeking to enhance their libido and deepen their intimate connection, recognizing and valuing individual differences in gender identity is a crucial step. It's about moving beyond surface-level attraction and tapping into the core of what makes us truly human. The journey of exploring gender identity within a relationship is not just about understanding your partner but is also about discovering more about yourself in the process.

At times, this exploration may require redefining what desire means within the relationship. For some, this might involve exploring new desires or re-evaluating existing ones, ensuring they're aligned with each partner's true self. Among the challenges that may arise, the commitment to respecting individual differences can serve as a guiding light, fostering resilience and adaptability in partnership.

Additionally, respecting individual differences aligns with creating an inclusive environment where every partner feels valued and respected. Inclusivity in relationships contributes to enhanced intimacy, as both partners feel secure enough to express their identities and desires fully. This openness can reignite passion that may have dimmed under societal or self-imposed pressures.

In essence, respecting individual differences widens the landscape of intimacy and desire, allowing couples to discover more vibrant ways to connect. This journey is as much about celebrating what makes us unique as it is about embracing the commonalities that bind us. Both partners stand to gain not only a renewed passion for each other but a renewed passion for themselves as well.

In your personal journey to enhance libido and deepen connection, remember the power that lies in respecting individual differences. It involves cultivating a space where both you and your partner can safely and authentically express who you are. Through this, intimacy can become not just a physical act but a profound union of souls, enriched by the full spectrum of human experience. As partners learn to cherish the unique qualities each brings to their relationship, they unlock the potential for genuine, lasting passion.

Ultimately, the tapestry of human connection becomes more intricate and beautiful when it includes every thread of identity and desire. Respecting individual differences propels us toward a fuller, more authentic experience of love and connection—one where desire isn't just reignited but burns brighter than ever.

Chapter 22:
The Role of Adventure and Novelty

Adventure and novelty have the power to invigorate the spirit and rejuvenate relationships by fostering anticipation and excitement. When couples embark on new experiences together, whether it be venturing into uncharted hobbies or exploring unfamiliar landscapes, they cultivate a sense of discovery and possibility. This shared journey not only strengthens bonds but also rekindles desire by creating an environment ripe for spontaneity and passion. The process of stepping out of the comfort zone and embracing the unknown can reignite the spark that routine might have dulled over time. As partners open themselves up to fun and adventurous dates, they break free from monotonous patterns, allowing their connections to evolve dynamically. It's this infusion of novelty that breathes fresh air into their intimate lives, making each moment feel as thrilling as the first. By prioritizing these novel experiences, couples create lasting memories that deepen their emotional and physical intimacy, paving the way for a more fulfilling and adventurous love life.

Trying New Activities Together

Embracing new activities as a couple is like opening a window to a fresh breeze of possibility and excitement. It involves stepping out of your comfort zones into a world where shared experiences can become the foundation of a deeper connection. Whether you're venturing into a hobby, exploring the outdoors, or trying a novel experience, the essence lies in engaging in something new together. The thrill and sometimes the challenge of the unknown can spark a sense of unity and ignite the passion that may have been dulled by routine.

The familiarity of the everyday can create a sense of security, but it often becomes the silent thief of adventure in relationships. Imagine the excitement of planning a weekend escape to somewhere you've never been, or even taking a class together in a skill neither of you has tried before. These activities offer more than just fun; they introduce elements of surprise and unpredictability, which are known to be adrenaline boosters. Shared adventures release dopamine, a feel-good hormone, fostering feelings of happiness and attraction.

Let's talk about interests. Discovering mutual interests or supporting each other's individual passions can create a bond that strengthens intimacy. For example, if one partner loves painting, the other could suggest attending an art class together. This not only provides support but also encourages engagement in the other's world. The experience of learning and improving alongside one another can fuel conversations and create memories that linger long after the paint has dried.

Now, consider activities that involve a bit of physicality or require working as a team—such as rock climbing, dancing, or even a cooking class. Shared accomplishments like reaching the top of a climbing wall can drive home personal and joint achievements, affirming mutual capabilities and trust. Team-oriented activities enhance communication and reliance on each other, qualities that are transferable to all aspects of the relationship.

Every relationship can benefit from a touch of the extraordinary. Planning an unusual date night or a weekend filled with spontaneous activities can revive the excitement of your early relationship days. Instead of the usual dinner and a movie, how about planning a scavenger hunt through the city or watching a meteor shower from a nearby field? The key is to infuse your time together with unique elements that provoke curiosity and exploration, this helps counteract monotony.

Couples who consistently try new activities are reported to have higher relationship satisfaction and better intimacy. This doesn't require a grand gesture or exhaustive planning. Start small. Try cooking a new recipe together or taking a different path during your evening walk. It's the openness to trying something new and the unpredictability it brings that fosters a shared sense of novelty.

Furthermore, trying new activities challenges you both individually and as a team. It forces you to pay attention to the present moment, enhancing awareness and mindfulness, which are fundamental in appreciating each other more deeply. The more you share these growth opportunities, the more you're likely to communicate effectively and understand each other's capabilities and thresholds.

Setting aside time to engage in novel experiences doesn't have to feel like a chore. Instead, think of it as an investment in your relationship's health. Allow yourself the freedom to let your guard down and laugh together; these are times when vulnerability is most powerful. Whether it's through laughter or within the shared silence of a moonlit hike, these moments count.

For those who crave adventure, traveling to somewhere unexplored by either of you could be the answer. Travel offers a multitude of new tastes, sights, and sounds, setting a table rich with opportunities to weave new stories into your relationship's fabric. The shared journey, with all its unexpected turns, can strengthen your team spirit and create an unspoken understanding.

Novel activities can also include small-scale adventures. How about mastering a new language together, one word at a time, or embarking on a photographic challenge capturing candid moments of shared light and shadow? These are shared journeys where progress is measured in laughter and the warmth of knowing glances.

Ultimately, trying new activities together is not just about having new conversations or stories to tell; it's about rediscovering the joy of your companion in a fresh context. The endeavor itself can refresh your outlook on partnership and intimacy—essentially making the familiar exciting once more. By reigniting the sense of curiosity and wonder, you continually nurture and refresh your connection, which is, at its core, the very essence of a robust and fulfilling relationship.

In creating these authentic experiences, you not only break the monotony; you pave the way for a deeper understanding of shared and individual identities, thus fostering love and connection that stand the test of time. So step out together, embrace the streak of newness, and look forward to the adventure each day can bring when you're open to seeing it as a beginning rather than an end.

Spicing Up Your Routine

Injecting a sense of adventure and novelty into your routine can make a significant difference in rekindling desire and building a deeper connection with your partner. In the whirlwind of daily life, routines can become monotonous, and the thrill of discovery often fades. By consciously planning fun and adventurous dates, you create shared experiences that break away from the usual patterns, inviting a fresh burst of energy into your relationship. It's about stepping out of your comfort zones and embracing the unexpected, whether it's trying a new dance class, exploring a different part of town together, or even recreating your first date with a twist. These moments offer an opportunity to see new facets of each other, sparking curiosity and a renewed sense of intimacy. In doing so, you not only enhance your libido but also nurture a bond that thrives on excitement, discovery, and love.

Fun and Adventurous Dates As we dive into the realm of keeping our relationships vibrant and alive, we find that introducing fun and adventurous dates can play a crucial role. These experiences not only break the monotony of daily routines but also infuse a sense of novelty and excitement into our lives. When we step outside our comfort zones with our partners, we open the door to shared experiences that are both exhilarating and bonding.

Imagine embarking on a spontaneous road trip to nowhere in particular. The open road, the thrill of the unknown, and the laughter shared over a roadside diner meal can build an adventure that strengthens connections. It's not just about the destination; it's about enjoying the journey together. Experiencing new things, whether they're as simple as trying an unfamiliar dish or as daring as surfing lessons, boosts the production of dopamine, the "feel-good" neurotransmitter. This can heighten both excitement and intimacy in your relationship.

For those who seek a touch of romance, consider a starlit picnic in your backyard or local park. The simplicity of laying on a blanket under the vast night sky, counting stars, or even spotting constellations ignites a sense of wonder and closeness. Pair this with a playlist of your shared favorite songs or simply the rustle of the breeze, and you create a memorable, romantic evening. Such intimate moments allow couples to engage in heartfelt conversations, deepening their emotional and physical connection.

If you're an adventurous pair craving a bit more thrill, how about indoor rock climbing? It's a fun way to challenge each other, offering a chance to support and encourage one another through every climb and descent. Safety gear ensures it's not as dangerous as it looks, and conquering those heights together can symbolize overcoming challenges in your relationship. The shared adrenaline and subsequent endorphin rush can create positive associations, reinforcing your bond.

For the more creatively inclined, taking a pottery or painting class together can be incredibly rewarding. Not only do you learn a new skill, but working with your hands alongside your partner can be grounding and therapeutic. As you create art, you're also crafting a shared narrative, filled with imperfections and unique beauty. Watching each other's process, the quirks, and intricacies of creating, can lead to a deeper understanding and appreciation for one another.

Spicing up your routine doesn't always require grand gestures or expensive outings. Sometimes, novelty can be found in the familiar turned unusual. For instance, planning a surprise tour in your own city can reveal hidden gems you've always overlooked. Becoming tourists in your own locale encourages curiosity and the pleasure of rediscovery. Whether it's visiting art installations, exploring nature reserves, or trying new restaurants, these mini-adventures revitalize the mundane.

If competing excites you, consider hosting a home-cooked meal challenge. Each partner can concoct a dish, and the whole process becomes a playful contest filled with love and laughter. This allows for friendly competition, creativity in the kitchen, and a shared meal that's filled with stories and surprises. It's these little moments of playful rivalry and shared indulgence that keep relationships lively.

At times, taking a step back from your routine is the change you need. Book a weekend cabin retreat, where technology is minimized, and nature is at its finest. Disconnecting from the digital world allows you to reconnect with each other. Walks in the forest, dips in the lake, or sitting by a roaring firelight leads to meaningful conversations and serenity that urban life often lacks. It's these breaks from the digital ties that bind us that help rediscover the essence of each other's presence.

For those nights when stepping out seems too much, transform your living room into a dance floor. Dim the lights, create a playlist of songs that chart your relationship's timeline, and dance. This spontaneous burst of movement and joy bridges the gap between routine and romance. It's about losing yourselves in each other's energy, feeling the music, and the closeness that dancing brings.

Ultimately, introducing fun and adventurous dates into your relationship is about being intentional and present. While these activities can be exciting, their true value lies in the time and attention you dedicate to each other. By making space for such adventures, you honor the space and closeness needed for a thriving connection. Each date becomes a chapter in your shared story, a story that continues to be written with spontaneity, love, and courage.

Consider these adventures a form of play—vital to adult relationships just as it is for children. Play fosters creativity, resilience, and a sense of aliveness that can rekindle passion. Let each event be a new exploration, undertaking every moment with enthusiasm and open heart. Your commitment to discovering joy in one another ensures that your love remains dynamic and fulfilling.

Novel Experiences add a spark to our routines, stirring something deep within us that yearns for the unexpected. It's this zest for the new that can weave a fresh tapestry of excitement into the fabric of our daily lives, especially when it comes to our intimate relationships. Imagine for a moment a life where every day felt exactly like the last, a monotonous cycle lacking variation or surprise. It's like watching your favorite movie on repeat; initially comforting, perhaps, but it eventually loses its edge. Now, layer that analogy over a romantic relationship. The mundane turns routine, fading the vibrancy of passion.

When partners consciously choose to introduce novel experiences into their shared lives, they engage in more than just mere escape from routine. It's a dance with vulnerability where each partner steps slightly into the unknown. This willingness to explore new territories together can forge formidable bonds of trust and intimacy. As they embark on these adventures, partners gaze across new vistas of possibility, seeing each other in lights perhaps never imagined before. And herein lies the magic: it's not always the destination of these experiences that matters most, but the journey—the unexpected revelations of each other that surface along the way.

Consider a couple taking a spontaneous road trip to an unfamiliar town, each bend in the road offers not just new landscapes, but opportunities for conversation and discovery they wouldn't normally have. During this journey, they may find joy in a hole-in-the-wall eatery, a hidden hiking trail, or even a roadside art gallery. These shared experiences enrich their narrative, layering new chapters with textures and colors beyond the monochrome of everyday existence.

In another scenario, novel experiences might manifest as something intimate and personal: cooking a new dish together. The clattering of pans, the sizzle of ingredients, and the aromatic symphony that fills the kitchen—all contribute to a sensory journey shared equally. A misstep might result in a burnt batch, yet even in these moments, laughter and intimacy are rekindled, far from the familiar dining choices or take-out habits. It's in these shared learning moments that partners grow closer, fostering a climate where candidness and creativity thrive.

However, the introduction of novelty should not be synonymous with the uncomfortable or unsafe. The idea is not to push boundaries recklessly but rather gently test them in ways that encourage mutual exploration and respect. Switch the perspective to a shared gym class or dance lesson, where learning a new skill becomes a bonding experience. The unfamiliarity of the steps or routine makes room for joint encouragement and even the occasional laughter at missed steps—all of which contribute to the cultivation of a kind and supportive environment.

It is essential to recognize that novelty can take diverse forms. It might be as grand as planning a surprise getaway or as simple as a twilight picnic in the backyard. While grand gestures have their place, often the smaller acts leave a lasting impact. Witnessing the sunrise together, visiting a local museum, or attending a community event can ignite sparks of discovery. These moments require attentive presence and open-mindedness, asking each partner to unveil parts of their hearts that had been perhaps hidden under life's ordinary pressures.

Furthermore, spicing up your routine with these experiences can rekindle aspects of attraction that have become subdued over time. The novelty has an invigorating quality, often reigniting the desire and playfulness that define the early stages of a relationship. With each new adventure embarked upon, a bank of shared memories is expanded, which in times can act as a foundation when faced with challenges in the relationship. They serve as reminders of what can be accomplished together, of the adventures that await just around the corner.

By incorporating regular elements of surprise or newness, couples can prevent their interactions from becoming stagnant. This practice encourages both partners to remain engaged and intrigued, constantly learning about one another in evolving ways. It underscores adventure as a critical factor in deepening intimacy—a pathway to more fulfilling connections where imagination and reality coalesce.

At the same time, it's crucial to remember that respect and communication underpin all novel experiences. Engaging in open dialogues about what types of adventures each partner is comfortable with strengthens the experience. Ensuring mutual consent and interest makes the adventure more enjoyable, removing any potential anxieties or pressures. The fabric of trust is strengthened through assured communication, manifesting an environment where innovative adventures become regular fixtures rather than rare exceptions.

Ultimately, by embracing novel experiences, couples glimpse the boundless horizons that love can traverse. They escape the confinements of predictability and sameness, guided instead by curiosity and wonder. As partners bravely stride into the uncharted, they learn anew not just about the world around them, but about themselves and each other. With every venture, with every shared shadow and light, they craft a narrative unique to their bond, making their journey through life together an adventure in its own right.

Chapter 23:
Long-Distance Relationship Challenges

Long-distance relationships, while challenging, don't have to mean the end of intimacy or desire. The key is finding creative ways to nurture the connection, even when miles apart. By embracing technology, couples can maintain a sense of closeness through heartfelt video calls and virtual dates that rekindle romance and deepen the bond. It's essential to establish open lines of communication, employing techniques such as shared daily recaps or sending surprise care packages filled with personal touches. These gestures go a long way in reducing the emotional distance. Understanding each other's love languages and regularly expressing appreciation can bolster emotional intimacy, transforming geographical separation into an opportunity for growth and renewed passion. With creativity and commitment, couples can maintain a dynamic emotional connection that fuels their desires, ensuring the flame of their relationship continues to burn brightly despite the distance.

Keeping Intimacy Alive Remotely

Long-distance relationships are a testament to the strength and resilience of the human heart. In a world divided by miles, keeping intimacy alive is both a challenge and an adventure. It's about finding ways to touch, to feel, and to connect even when touch isn't physically possible. With a blend of invention, communication, and emotional depth, couples can transcend the barriers of distance and cultivate a deep, passionate connection that thrives despite the miles.

Emotional intimacy is the cornerstone of any relationship, but it becomes even more critical in a long-distance setting where physical closeness is absent. It's about building a bridge of shared experiences and conversations that are as vivid and touching as a tender kiss. Couples can use music to create shared playlists that evoke shared feelings and memories, listen to podcasts together, or watch movies at the same time and share their reactions.

One of the keys to keeping the flame alive is to invest in meaningful communication tools. Messaging and video chatting services offer a convenient means to maintain communication, reducing the sense of separation. But beyond the convenience, they invite a chance to be present for each other. Dedicate time, even if it's just a few moments each morning or before sleep, to engage in a conversation that delves deeper than the surface level.

Beyond conversations, sharing daily routines and little moments can foster intimacy. Simple acts like video calling each morning for coffee or sharing photos of moments throughout the day draw partners into each other's lives. This regular sharing weaves a tapestry of genuine connection that carries more significance than grand gestures might.

Creating routines and rituals is another way to bridge the gap. This process might include scheduling regular visits, where possible, and planning future activities can give partners something to look forward to. The anticipation of reuniting not only strengthens the bond but also provides a sense of stability and commitment as you navigate the hurdles of separation.

Personalized tokens of affection are lovely surprises that keep the romance alive. Write handwritten letters, send personalized gifts that express fond memories, or create a journal where you each pen down thoughts and elaborate on shared dreams. These tangible reminders of love can fill empty spaces with warmth and anticipation.

The digital age offers a unique playground for creativity. Virtual reality (VR) technology, for example, can allow couples to explore distant lands together or meet in virtual spaces. Although it may sound futuristic, VR can simulate shared experiences, offering a glimpse of shared realities that's otherwise challenging to accomplish from afar.

Even traditional methods can take a digital twist—online games have evolved to become social as well as fun. Logging in and playing together can be an engaging way to spend time, whether politically strategizing in a massive multiplayer game or banding together on a cooperative quest.

And when the longing becomes challenging to bear, expressing vulnerability and longing to be together is perfectly natural. Acknowledging feelings of loneliness and yearning can foster understanding. It's a way of feeling each other's presence through words and emotions, offering comfort and encouragement.

It's equally important to close the gap by planning casual "dates." From virtual cooking classes where you each whip up a meal in your kitchen, to artistic sessions where couples paint or draw what they imagine the other might be doing, these events bolster a sense of partnership and fun. They help maintain a semblance of normalcy and cultivation of mutual hobbies, planting seeds for shared futures.

Every couple is different, and what works for one might not work for all. Some might thrive on daily video calls, while others cherish watching the same television show while texting commentary in real-time. The secret lies in understanding each other's needs and striving to meet them in thoughtful, imaginative ways.

All challenges of long-distance relationships can be viewed as opportunities for growth and creativity. Keeping intimacy alive remotely isn't about simply surviving but thriving through love. It's about forging connections filled with joy and weathering challenges with courage while the boundaries of physical absence fade away into insignificance.

And amidst the vast world that separates, it's in these shared moments that partners discover a universe entirely their own, woven from heartstrings, whispered dreams, and an unwavering bond that refuses to acknowledge distance. As they navigate this shared journey, they create a love story that stands as a testament to the enduring power of love—a beacon of passion shining brightly across miles.

Creative Solutions for Connection

In long-distance relationships, maintaining a meaningful connection can be both challenging and rewarding, encouraging partners to think outside the box and get creative with their interactions. A myriad of virtual activities can foster intimacy from afar: consider setting up virtual date nights where you explore new recipes together, watch a movie simultaneously, or play interactive online games. These shared experiences not only bring joy but also cultivate a sense of togetherness and collaboration. Spice things up by sending thoughtful surprise packages that reflect shared interests or cherished memories, or indulge in handwritten love letters to deepen emotional connections. Video calls can be made more intimate by setting the ambiance with candles and music, simulating a shared physical space that's comforting and familiar. By embracing technology and viewing the distance as an opportunity for creativity rather than a limitation, couples can nurture their bond, strengthening the fabric of their relationship despite the miles that separate them.

Virtual Date Ideas embrace the magic of blending technology with intimacy to bridge the distance that often challenges long-distance relationships. In the realm of romance, creativity becomes your biggest ally, offering a plethora of ways to nurture connection even when miles apart. It's about bringing your worlds closer together, crafting moments where love isn't just spoken but felt deeply across screens.

Imagine an evening where the two of you explore virtual travel. Platforms dedicated to virtual reality tours can whisk you both away to iconic landmarks around the globe. Together, you could explore the grandeur of Paris at sunset or the ancient streets of Rome. Each click is not just an adventure but an opportunity to learn more about each other's interests and dream destinations, building anticipation for that day when you might visit in person.

For a more intimate setting, consider hosting a virtual movie night. Simply select a movie or series, sync your viewing using platforms that allow simultaneous watching, and snuggle up with your favorite snacks. Interact freely during the movie, exchanging thoughts, jokes, and perhaps a shared sigh during romantic scenes. These nights can end with discussions extending into the wee hours, further deepening your bond.

Cooking is another delightful virtual date idea. Decide on a recipe, shop for ingredients, and cook 'together' over a video call. This shared experience not only hones your culinary skills but also strengthens your sense of partnership. Plus, there's laughter in the chaos of kitchen mishaps, and joy when you unveil your creations, making it an exciting and interactive affair.

For those who cherish intellectual bonding, a virtual book club can be a great fit. Choose a book to read individually and set a date to discuss it. The discussions can spark insightful conversations, reveal new perspectives, and pave the way for philosophical exchanges. This not only nurtures emotional intimacy but intellectual satisfaction as well, adding layers to your relationship.

Interactive games also offer a playful dimension to virtual dating. Whether it's solving puzzles in an online escape room, embarking on adventures in multiplayer games, or even playing a simple game of chess, the time you spend playing together reinforces teamwork and light-hearted competition, all the while keeping the fun alive.

For those special evenings when you both crave tranquility, you might consider a virtual stargazing date. Download an astronomy app, gaze at the stars from your respective locations, and identify constellations together. There's something profoundly romantic about lying under the same sky, discussing the mysteries of the universe, and dreaming together in a moment of quietude.

Don't underestimate the power of a simple call where you play music for each other. Music has the unique ability to evoke emotions, and sharing favorite tunes can become a moving experience, uncovering memories and feelings, and enabling mutual vulnerability. Create a playlist together that symbolizes your journey, adding songs that define different phases of your relationship.

Virtual art classes can also serve as an exciting date option. Choose a class, gather your art supplies, and let the creativity flow. Share your creations at the end, laugh at the inevitable imperfections, and admire each other's expressive strokes. It's a wonderful way to explore new sides of each other and foster artistic appreciation.

Then there are personalized quizzes meant to test your knowledge of each other. You can amuse yourselves with questions about your likes, dislikes, trivia about memorable moments you've shared, or even future aspirations. Such quizzes spark conversations, uncover forgotten memories, and maybe even reveal unknown facets about each other.

Lastly, let's not forget the intimacy of planning the future. Dedicate time to dream and plan about your visits, future home, or shared goals. Create vision boards digitally, share your hopes and dreams, and reinforce the belief that the distance is temporary, further fortifying your commitment to what lies ahead.

In the end, the spirit of these virtual date ideas lies not just in the activities themselves but in the intent to maintain and deepen connection. By embracing creativity and open communication, you not only tackle the challenges of distance but turn them into opportunities to learn, grow, and love more profoundly. The distance, while a trial, becomes an intricate part of your love story—one where each chapter is filled with evidence of your resilience and commitment.

Communication Techniques are indispensable in maintaining intimacy within long-distance relationships, offering creative solutions to bridge the physical gap between partners. The absence of physical presence might seem daunting, but through effective communication, it can serve as an opportunity to deepen emotional connections. By leveraging a combination of verbal and non-verbal cues, couples can transcend the constraints of distance and nurture their bond with authenticity and intimacy.

Beginning with the simplest tool in our conversational arsenal— words. Words can build bridges over the longest miles. Regular, meaningful dialogue is key to keeping the spark alive; it's not just about frequency but also about depth and quality. Engaging in conversations that delve into each other's aspirations, worries, and dreams offers an introspective exchange that mimics the closeness of being together. As each partner shares their inner world, a tapestry of mutual understanding and emotional resonance is woven.

Acknowledging that tone and timing are as important as the message itself is critical. When communicating across time zones, being considerate of each other's schedules can prevent misunderstandings and foster a respectful communication rhythm. Plus, understanding how one's mood and tone can drastically alter a message's reception is crucial. Keeping a compassionate and thoughtful approach can make all the difference in navigating challenging conversations.

Though words are powerful, silence can also speak volumes—or whispers, at least, in the language of love. Silence interspersed with meaningful pauses allows for reflection and anticipation, creating a rhythm akin to a dance choreographed just for two. It adds depth to conversations and ensures that moments of solitude are not mistaken for neglect but rather opportunities to contemplate and appreciate the exchange.

Technology ushers in an array of possibilities for non-verbal communication that can enhance your connection creatively. Consider exchanging photos, videos, or voice notes that capture not just moments but emotions. A candid image or the sound of your partner's laughter can evoke a sense of presence and immediacy, captivating the heart more vividly than mere text. These snippets of everyday life simulate the shared space that a physical relationship naturally enjoys.

Video calls present yet another realm for authentic connection. Beyond mere chats, these calls offer the ability to "see" each other regularly, which can simulate a face-to-face interaction. A great way to make these video interactions more intimate is by creating shared rituals, like cooking the same meal together or watching a movie simultaneously. These shared experiences can transport the mundane into memorable, bonding activities.

A delightful and often underestimated form of communication is letter writing. The tangible and personal nature of letters endows them with a quaint charm, serving as intimate tokens of affection. Unlike instant messaging, letters capture a snapshot of one's feelings in a particular moment, preserved on paper, creating a lasting testament of the relationship's journey.

Effective communication thrives on sincerity. Authentic expressions of love and affection, whether spoken or written, should convey genuine emotions. Authenticity requires vulnerability; it invites partners to reveal themselves without guise or guard, weaving trust into the fabric of the relationship. This openness can fortify the emotional intimacy crucial for thriving long-distance partnerships.

Creative communication is not without challenges, and maintaining enthusiasm and innovation is essential as months stretch into years. Changing up your communication methods and experimenting with different ways to connect can keep the experience invigorating. Whether it's starting a shared blog, crafting a travel plan wishlist, or sending personalized playlists, the key is to keep the connection dynamic and evolving, just like a living entity.

Finally, never underestimate the power of small tokens of affection delivered in creative ways. From surprise hand-delivered gifts to spontaneously ordered dinner over the likes of apps, these gestures illustrate thoughtfulness and attentiveness, lending a tangible presence to intangible communication. Importantly, these actions remind partners that, although apart, their relationship remains a priority and a source of joy and sustenance.

Ultimately, communication techniques in long-distance relationships are about transcending the physical separation with emotional closeness. The art of listening, expressing, and creatively connecting is central to converting this geographical gap into a landscape of love and understanding. When nurtured with care and creativity, distance transforms into a canvas upon which partners paint their unique version of intimacy, painting with words, gestures, and shared dreams.

Chapter 24:
Reconnecting After a
Breakup or Crisis

In the delicate dance of reconnection, healing and rekindling passion after a breakup or crisis can feel both daunting and invigorating. As the heart navigates the labyrinth of past hurts and future hopes, there's an undeniable beauty in the possibility of a renewed partnership. When trust has been bruised, taking deliberate steps towards rebuilding it can facilitate a fresh start. To embrace this journey, it's vital to acknowledge and process grief and loss; allowing these emotions to ebb and flow opens the pathway to moving forward. Couples may find strength in shared vulnerability, where communication fosters deeper understanding and ignites the flickering embers of desire. It's about crafting strategies that not only mend the fragile seams of the relationship but also weave new threads of love and intimacy, transforming challenges into opportunities for growth and closeness.

Healing and Rekindling Passion

In the journey of love, relationships can sometimes endure turbulence, leading to periods of separation or crisis. The path to healing and rekindling passion begins with understanding that it's a process—a delicate one that requires patience, commitment, and openness to change.

Actively working on re-establishing intimacy after a breakup or crisis can be both challenging and rewarding. This phase doesn't just involve smoothing over past grievances but actively working towards building a stronger foundation. It's essential to acknowledge that both partners may bring unresolved emotions into the reconciliatory process. These feelings need to be aired compassionately and constructively.

Open and honest discussions are cornerstones of reigniting passion. It's within these conversations that hidden desires and longings can emerge, allowing both partners to address them. Sharing insights about past experiences, what brings joy, or what might have been missing in the relationship can lead to a new, shared understanding.

Rekindling passion also involves rekindling the individual spark within oneself. It's important to foster a strong sense of self-love and individual wellbeing. When one takes steps to care for their physical and emotional health, it brings a more vibrant energy into the relationship. This is the empowerment that gives way for shared intimacy to flourish anew.

Often, couples find that introducing new experiences into their relationship ignites a sense of adventure and novelty. It may involve trying new activities together, visiting places previously unexplored, or engaging in new hobbies. This infusion of novelty revitalizes the relationship and opens avenues for deeper emotional and physical connections.

Alongside adventure, integrating small, meaningful gestures of love into daily interactions can help maintain and deepen intimacy. These don't have to be grand. Simple acts, such as cooking a favorite meal, sharing a heartfelt note, or planning a spontaneous outing, can communicate love and appreciation, ultimately fortifying the relationship's bond.

Rekindling passion also entails physical reconnection, which can be achieved through the power of touch and closeness. Engaging in sensual practices, such as massage, or simply spending time in physical proximity can rekindle the sensory memories of affection and affinity. Embracing each other's presence brings warmth and assures that vulnerability is safe and welcome.

For reconciliation to succeed, addressing past breaches of trust is crucial. Both partners must commit to honesty and transparency, laying all feelings bare. Apologies, when given without reservation, lay the groundwork for forgiveness and acceptance. It takes time and effort for trust to rebuild, but every step taken together counts immensely.

During this journey, it's important to remember that setbacks may occur. Navigating through these obstacles demands resilience and understanding. Couples should seek common goals for their relationship, creating a shared vision of their future that includes mutual support and growth. This shared vision acts as a guiding star, keeping them focused on what truly matters and helping them navigate turbulent times.

Ultimately, healing and rekindling passion after a breakup or crisis is an act of courage and love. It demands that both partners commit to moving forward with a spirit of rebuilding a connection that was once thought broken. It invites an opportunity for discovering depths and heights of love and intimacy they might not have previously imagined.

This period in the relationships is not merely about mending the past, but about embarking on a journey together with renewed appreciation and admiration for each other. It's a celebration of resilience—a testament to the power of love and its ability to overcome hardship and flourish in new, extraordinary ways.

Steps for Rebuilding Trust

Rebuilding trust after a breakup or crisis requires a delicate yet determined approach. Begin by acknowledging past mistakes and communicating openly with your partner about your intentions to mend the relationship. It's crucial to be patient, as trust is rebuilt over time through consistent actions that demonstrate commitment and honesty. Taking small, thoughtful steps can help re-establish a foundation of trust, such as setting clear expectations and being reliable in fulfilling promises. Encourage vulnerability by creating a safe space where both partners can express their feelings without fear of judgment. As you navigate this healing journey, remember that trust is not merely a destination but a continual practice of empathy, understanding, and connection that strengthens your intimacy and renews the passion in your shared life together.

Navigating Grief and Loss explores the challenging terrain of emotions that come with the end of a relationship or a significant life crisis, intricately tied to the journey of rebuilding trust. Such experiences can shake the very foundation of your emotional wellbeing, leaving a sense of emptiness that can seem insurmountable. Yet, it is vital to acknowledge that these feelings, as intense and overwhelming as they may be, are a normal part of the healing process. Loss, in any form, can complicate the path to restoring faith in your partner and yourself, but embracing the grieving process is essential to moving forward. Grief uniquely affects each individual, and understanding this personal journey is crucial to bridging the gap left by past events.

One of the first steps in healing is allowing yourself to feel. Often, there is an urge to suppress emotions to avoid pain, but acknowledging sorrow and disappointment is important for genuine recovery. Bottling up grief can lead to emotional blockages that hinder the resurrection of trust. Instead, create space for these emotions, allowing yourself to feel them fully and find lessons within them. Journaling can be a powerful tool here, providing a safe outlet to express whatever arises. Writing about your thoughts and emotions helps in processing the chaos that often accompanies grief and loss. It can facilitate a deeper understanding of personal needs and desires, laying the groundwork for rebuilding trust.

Communication with yourself and your partner plays a pivotal role in reconnecting after experiencing grief and loss. Establishing an open dialogue can offer insights into each other's vulnerabilities and fears, fostering an environment where trust can slowly regrow. This dialogue doesn't have to be perfect or follow a strict format; it just needs to be honest. By sharing your feelings of grief and the impact it has had, you encourage your partner to do the same. This mutual exchange not only strengthens your emotional bond but also opens pathways to empathy, which is integral to trust rebuilding.

As you navigate through this journey, patience becomes your greatest ally. Trust, once fractured by grief or crisis, needs time to heal. It's a gradual process where small, consistent actions build towards restoring what was lost. Each step taken together, no matter how minor, can help to weave a new fabric of trust. Focus on small gestures, such as maintaining eye contact, active listening, and affirming each other's feelings. Together, these steps form the foundation upon which trust can be rebuilt, supporting the larger goal of rekindling deep desire and connection.

Furthermore, incorporating rituals or routines that signify new beginnings can be beneficial. Creating rituals—like a weekly check-in session where both of you discuss your emotional states or aspirations—can act as anchors, grounding your relationship amidst the instability that grief can bring. It's not about rigid structures but rather about finding moments that honor both of your journeys.

These rituals serve as gentle reminders of progress and commitment to healing, nurturing the trust that sustains your intimate connection.

Grappling with grief can sometimes feel like a solitary endeavor, but recognizing that you are not alone is crucial. Engage with support systems outside of the relationship, like friendships, family, or professional counseling. These connections provide external perspectives that can help you manage your emotions and reinforce your resilience. Counselors, specifically, can offer guidance tailored to your unique circumstances, allowing you to explore emotions deeply, which might otherwise remain unexamined when left solely to self-reflection.

Through these external engagements, you can gather fresh insights and coping mechanisms that can actively contribute to rebuilding personal and shared trust. Leaning on others for support doesn't diminish the bond between you and your partner; rather, it strengthens it by ensuring you're both emotionally equipped to participate fully in the relationship.

Building trust after a significant crisis or breakup involves a conscious commitment to change. It's a mutual endeavor that invites both partners to reflect, adapt, and rediscover one another. The wounds inflicted by grief, while initially daunting, can become a guiding force toward transformative healing within your relationship. As you navigate this terrain, remember that the journey itself can enhance your empathy and compassion, ultimately fostering a more profound connection.

In the end, navigating grief and loss is not about forgetting the past but about integrating experiences into the tapestry of your shared life. It's about allowing these experiences to inform your growth and bring you closer together in understanding and love. From the ashes of loss, new possibilities for trust and connection can emerge, revitalizing your relationship. With careful navigation, patience, and open-heartedness, the chapters of grief can turn into a story of resilience and strengthened intimacy.

As you continue to heal and rebuild, celebrate the small victories along the way. These moments, though often understated, signify the return of hope and faith in your partnership. Reestablishing trust after grief necessitates vulnerability, but in that vulnerability lies the potential for profound renewal and an enduring connection that once again binds your hearts together. Understanding and compassion become your compass, guiding you towards the deeper intimacy and trust you both seek.

Strategies for Moving Forward offer a pathway to a renewed sense of connection and intimacy after the upheaval of a breakup or personal crisis. Life's setbacks can leave us feeling disconnected or wary, but they also provide opportunities to rebuild and strengthen the foundation of our relationships. By focusing on intentional actions and open communication, couples can nurture their bond with empathy and understanding, ultimately reigniting the flame of desire and passion.

First and foremost, acknowledge that healing takes time. Rushing this process could result in unresolved emotions or misunderstandings, leading to further disconnection. Give both yourself and your partner the grace of time to process past events. During this period, focus on personal reflection. Understand your feelings and identify the aspects of the past that need closure. This introspective journey is essential before coming together to move forward as a unit.

A crucial step in moving forward is open and honest communication. Create a safe space where both partners can express their thoughts, fears, and aspirations. These conversations should be devoid of judgment, and each partner must approach the dialogue with the willingness to listen and empathize. Practicing active listening can deepen understanding and foster a supportive environment, laying the groundwork for trust to flourish anew.

Developing new rituals can serve as an antidote to past hurts. By establishing fresh routines or traditions, couples can redefine their relationship dynamics. These rituals, whether it's a shared hobby or regular date nights, should be enjoyable and promote bonding. Think of these as the threads weaving a new tapestry of shared experiences, bringing couples closer than before.

Rebuilding trust isn't a monolithic task. It's achieved through a series of small, consistent actions. These may include making and keeping promises, demonstrating reliability in everyday situations, and showing gratitude. Expressing appreciation for each other daily strengthens your emotional connection and guards against the complacency that can erode trust over time.

An essential component of trust is accountability. Acknowledging past mistakes and demonstrating a commitment to change signals maturity and respect for the relationship. When one partner takes responsibility, it allows the other to feel seen and heard, building confidence in the renewed relationship. This step, though challenging, is critical for healing and growth.

Exploring vulnerabilities together can be transformative. Sharing deeply personal concerns and aspirations can deepen intimacy, reminding each partner of the unique bond they share. This process requires bravery and a readiness to lean into emotional discomfort, but it's often where the greatest growth and connection can occur. With openness, these shared moments become a testament to your journey together, fostering a resilient partnership.

Embrace the healing power of touch. A simple act like a reassuring hug can diminish stress and reinforce emotional bonds. Consider incorporating sensory experiences like giving each other massages or practicing mindful breathing exercises. Such physical connections often communicate what words cannot, enhancing emotional intimacy and rebuilding trust.

As your relationship progresses, focus on setting joint goals. Collaboratively setting intentions for your future embodies the commitment to move forward. These goals do not have to be grand; they can be as simple as trying new activities or achieving shared milestones. This forward-thinking approach keeps the relationship dynamic and aligned with your shared vision.

Remember that setbacks are a part of any relationship journey. Addressing problems promptly with empathy ensures they don't fester and disrupt the healing process. This steadfast approach emphasizes your commitment to building a constructive and loving future together. Resilience arises from facing challenges head-on and utilizing them as stepping stones toward deeper connection.

Lastly, don't underestimate the power of external support. Sometimes, an outside perspective can provide clarity and context. Couples therapy or individual counseling offers a structured environment to explore complex emotions, fostering growth and development. Professionals can guide you in areas like effective communication, conflict resolution, or rebuilding intimacy.

By weaving these strategies into the fabric of your relationship, you embrace the journey toward a revitalized connection. The path may not always be linear, but with patience and intentional effort, each step forward builds a strong fortress of love and trust, reigniting the desire and passion that initially brought you together.

Chapter 25:
Celebrating Love and Milestones

As couples journey through the tapestry of life together, it is these shared milestones and celebrations that stitch their stories with vibrant threads. Recognizing achievements as a team not only reinforces the bond you share but also infuses your relationship with renewed passion and commitment. Whether it's marking the success of a personal goal, an anniversary, or simply the joy of being together, planning these moments with intention creates rich, enduring memories. In the ebb and flow of daily life, such celebrations become sanctuaries of happiness, allowing partners to reflect, appreciate, and dream anew. By embracing and cherishing these junctures, you reaffirm the love and dedication that brought you together, paving the way for a future filled with love, connection, and shared achievements.

Recognizing Achievements Together

In the journey of love and life, milestones serve as both markers of progress and points of reflection. They stand as beautiful reminders of where two people have ventured together, in harmony and support, celebrating not just the achievements themselves but the shared effort to reach them.

Every relationship is a tapestry woven from experiences, successes, and even challenges. Recognizing achievements together means taking the time to do exactly that—to pause, acknowledge, and celebrate those very threads. It isn't solely about the grand gestures or monumental accomplishments but also the seemingly small victories that sustain and nourish a partnership. Perhaps it's as simple as successfully working together through a tumultuous week or as ambitious as achieving a long-discussed career goal or personal dream. The essence lies in the mutual recognition of what it has taken to arrive at this point, hand in hand.

Acknowledgement of these shared victories can reinvigorate desire and strengthen intimacy by reinforcing the bond between partners. This isn't merely ceremonial; it's an act of love, a reaffirmation that says, "We did this, together." So, embracing these celebrations can bring couples closer, strengthening the emotional and physical components of their relationship.

The power of shared acknowledgment lies in its ability to reinforce positive behavior and commitment within relationships. When partners come together to celebrate an achievement, they are also affirming the values they've cultivated together—teamwork, resilience, patience. In doing so, they are nurturing the desire to continue striving and growing as a unit.

Consider the variety of life events that may call for celebration: promotions, anniversaries, overcoming a particular challenge, or even more personal achievements like a health milestone or a creative accomplishment. The recognition of these milestones should be as diverse as the relationships they celebrate. For some, an impromptu date night might be the perfect acknowledgment; for others, a getaway or a simple heartfelt note might carry more weight. What's vital is the attention to the uniqueness these celebrations bring into one's lives.

Starting with an open dialogue about what milestones mean to each partner is fundamental. Each person might prioritize different achievements, and understanding that can aid in creating meaningful celebrations. This dialogue fosters emotional intimacy by allowing partners to express appreciation, hopes, and dreams, forming a deeper understanding of each other's values and aspirations.

Remember, celebrating achievements shouldn't become a source of pressure or competition. Instead, it should be an opportunity to reaffirm love and partnership. The celebrations are not about external validation but rather the internal satisfaction and connection they can generate. By removing expectations and focusing on the joy of shared accomplishment, partners can enjoy these moments fully.

Once these foundational conversations are in place, it may be helpful to set intentions for recognizing future achievements. Think of these as traditions or rituals that bind the relationship's fabric tighter. Whether it's committing to a monthly reflection on what's been accomplished or designing a personal 'celebration' space at home filled with mementos and memories that tell your unique story, these practices can enhance connection and commitment.

Furthermore, these recognitions play a crucial role in supporting each partner's individual growth. While celebrating together solidifies the partnership, acknowledging personal achievements within that framework allows both individuals to feel seen and supported. This dual celebration fosters an environment where each person's dreams are valued, contributing to a balanced relationship where both partners thrive.

Maintaining balance in celebrating is key. Ensure that recognition is genuine and balanced, avoiding any feelings of inequality or neglect. It's important to listen, adapt, and create a culture of mutual appreciation and validation. This not only enhances libido by creating a supportive, affirming environment but also maintains the partnership's long-term health and happiness.

The end goal of recognizing achievements together isn't just the moments themselves but the lasting bond they create. These moments, when cherished, become treasured memories that lay the foundation for a lifetime of shared dreams and aspirations. In revisiting these achievements, partners can draw strength, understanding, and compassion that bolster their everyday struggles and triumphs.

The act of recognizing achievements together is an investment in the future, an acknowledgment of the path you've walked, and a pledge towards the path yet to come. It's a celebration of not just what has been done, but who you are as partners—brave, united, and in love. May these shared celebrations fuel your journey towards a fulfilling and lasting connection.

Creating Long-Lasting Memories

Creating long-lasting memories with your partner is an art that blossoms from shared experiences and heartfelt gestures, weaving moments of joy and intimacy into the fabric of your relationship. When you celebrate life's milestones together, whether they're grand achievements or small victories, you lay down the foundation of a love story rich with reminiscences. It's about finding moments to pause, to cherish the bond you share, and to mark the passage of time with meaningful traditions or spontaneous adventures. Whether you're revisiting the place of your first date or embarking on a new journey together, these memories serve as enduring keepsakes, nurturing the passion that ignites your shared life. By consciously crafting these memories, you not only honor your partner but also fortify the connection that makes every moment together truly unforgettable.

Planning Celebrations is an integral practice in the art of creating long-lasting memories within your relationship. Imagine the joy and connection that arise when you and your partner take the time to plan celebrations that speak directly to your shared experiences and milestones — it's a powerful way to affirm your love and dedication to one another. Whether you're commemorating a wedding anniversary, the success of a challenging project, or even just the sheer gratitude for having found each other, each moment can be infused with a sense of wonder and intimacy that transcends the ordinary.

Often, the most memorable celebrations are those that reflect the distinctive nuances of your relationship. As you embark on planning these milestones, consider the interests and shared dreams that make your relationship unique. Perhaps it's an intimate dinner prepared together at home, a weekend getaway to a destination you've both longed to explore, or a surprise event crafted around a hobby or passion that you both cherish. Use your creativity to breathe life into the celebration, ensuring it becomes a tapestry of shared experiences and emotions.

A hallmark of unforgettable celebrations is the presence of surprises and personalized touches that resonate deeply. These can range from writing heartfelt letters or poems to creating a personalized playlist of songs that hold special meaning for you both. Such thoughtful gestures create a tapestry of intimacy and connection that can't be easily replicated. You may also consider inviting close friends or family to share in the joy, adding layers of shared history and support that amplify the occasion's significance.

Planning a celebration doesn't necessarily mean extravagant or costly events. The essence lies in the thoughtfulness and intention behind the gesture. Simplicity often carries more weight than grand exhibitions. Think of a quiet picnic in the park, a curated movie night with films that marked different stages of your relationship, or a walk down memory lane revisiting the locations that hold sentimental value. These intimate yet powerful moments can demonstrate to your partner that your love remains vibrant and attentive.

While spontaneity can provide excitement, a well-planned celebration ensures you both have space to anticipate and savor the event. Start by setting a date that honors the particular milestone you're celebrating. Consider each other's schedules and preferences to ensure the event feels relaxed and enjoyable rather than rushed or inconvenient. As the day approaches, the shared excitement builds a sense of anticipation, fostering connection even before the celebration begins.

Integrating rituals or traditions into your celebrations can imbue them with a sense of continuity and depth. Some couples find joy in recreating elements from past celebrations, adding new layers of meaning over the years. For instance, revisiting the location of your first date, or lighting a candle to mark the passing of each year together, can become cherished rituals that strengthen your bond over time. These repeated actions foster a narrative of togetherness that weaves through the fabric of your relationship.

Another dimension to consider while planning these celebrations involves future aspirations and dreams. While you're honoring the past, you can also use the occasion to articulate your future dreams and goals as a couple. This adds a proactive layer to the celebration, underlining the commitment you both share towards mutual growth and exploration. Writing down shared aspirations for the coming years, or incorporating vision boards into your day, can make the occasion an inspiring catalyst for both of you.

But planning doesn't just stop at ideas and execution — reflecting on the celebration afterward can enrich it further. Take time together to reminisce, sharing your favorite moments and recounting the feelings the event evoked. This reinforces the positive emotions and memories and sets a precedent for appreciating and valuing each event you share.

Importantly, remember that not all milestones will be happy or celebratory in the conventional sense. Some might be commemorations of overcoming adversity or surviving tough times together. In these instances, planning a celebration around resilience and strength can become a powerful tribute to your shared journey. It acknowledges the challenges you've faced while celebrating the unwavering partnership that helped you surmount them.

In summary, planning celebrations within a relationship is as much about the journey as the destination. It's about consciously creating a space where intimacy, gratitude, and shared joy thrive. By infusing your celebrations with authenticity, mutual preferences, and hopeful visions for the future, you cement these moments as lasting memories that you'll carry forward with love and affection for years to come.

Marking Important Dates is a sacred ritual that breathes life into the narrative of our shared journey, a practice that not only nurtures love but also reinforces the bonds that tie us to one another. In a world brimming with distractions, it is the mindful acknowledgment and celebration of these milestones that carve out spaces for connection. The act of remembering, of consciously marking a day, signifies its importance and the emotions tied to it. Whether it's a first date anniversary, a wedding, or the day you took that leap of trust to meet each other's families, these dates form the fabric of shared stories, unique only to you both.

When we celebrate these important dates, each moment becomes a chapter in the book of life you write together. Consider how you felt on the day you met; the exhilaration, the nervous anticipation, the tentative joy. Reverting to these moments, even if briefly, helps in rekindling the spark that's intertwined with the essence of your bond. It's more than just a celebration of an event; it's about savoring the love and growth experienced since then. It's a pause to appreciate one another and a reaffirmation of your journey together.

Marking important dates doesn't have to be grandiose or expensive. Sometimes, the simplicity of a handwritten note, an unexpected bouquet, or preparing a favorite meal is enough to say, "I remember; I cherish us." The beauty of these gestures lies in their sincerity. They convey that you are thoughtful, that you care enough to pause, remember, and act. It is these seemingly small acts that, over time, create a tapestry rich with memories and meaning.

At the heart of marking important dates is the desire to create a ritualistic anchoring point. It offers stability and predictability amidst life's ever-shifting tides. Rituals cultivate a rhythm that both partners come to anticipate with fondness and nostalgia. Over time, these become traditions that hold emotional weight. They are handy when life throws curveballs or during periods when it's tough to find time for each other. The traditions you build along the way serve as a consistent reminder of the foundation of love and togetherness you've established.

Engage in marking important dates as a team. Sit down together and reflect on which dates hold significance in your story. It might surprise you how each person recalls something special and different, showcasing the depth of your shared experiences. This collective reflection not only acknowledges the past but also sets a hopeful gaze towards the future. It's a conversation that fosters openness and understanding, qualities vital for a healthy and vibrant relationship.

Consider broadening the scope of these celebrations to include 'smaller' but meaningful moments: your first road trip, a movie night when you stayed up until dawn talking about dreams, or perhaps a hobby embarked upon together. For each couple, these mini-milestones offer cherished memories that remind both individuals of their shared life and how far they've come together. In this light, marking important dates becomes less about the calendar and more about the heart.

Technology, while often seen as a distraction, can be a useful ally in this venture. Simple tools like calendar reminders or planning apps can help ensure that these special dates are never overlooked. But remember, being alerted by a ding on your phone isn't as loving or impactful as genuinely committing a date to heart. Let the reminder serve as a prompt, but let your daily actions breathe life into the moment.

The celebration of important dates should not become a pressure point. The authenticity of your intent matters more than the execution. It's better to do something small and meaningful than to overextend financially or emotionally. If one partner is anxious about grand gestures, encourage them to embrace what feels natural and sincere. The essence lies in the shared memory and the laughter, tears, or quiet companionship that accompany it.

Finally, let these moments be opportunities for renewal. Each marked date should serve as a reminder of the love that persists and grows. It's a time to express gratitude, to look into your partner's eyes and reaffirm your commitment, your love, your companionship. Use these moments to recharge your emotional batteries, to reassure one another, and to plant seeds for the future. Celebrate the past, cherish the present, and dream about the possibilities that lie ahead.

In essence, marking important dates as part of "Creating Long-Lasting Memories" in your journey doesn't just honor where you've been, but also illuminates the path to where you are going. It's a commitment to continual growth and understanding, ensuring that your bond remains strong and vibrant. So, don't just mark the dates on your calendars; mark them in your hearts and let each one be a stepping stone towards deeper love and connection.

Conclusion

As we reach the conclusion of our exploration into enhancing libido and deepening intimacy, it's vital to reflect on the transformative journey we've undertaken together. Each step has not only illuminated a path towards understanding the intricate dance between passion and desire but has also empowered us with actionable insights to cultivate a fulfilling love life. The synergy between knowledge and action is where real change takes root, and it's this combination that can revive and reinvigorate connections.

Throughout this book, we've ventured into the scientific and emotional landscapes of desire, uncovering the truths that lie beneath common myths. We've learned that open dialogue and effective communication are the lifelines of vibrant relationships, establishing a foundation of trust and understanding. By engaging in conversations that matter, partners can navigate both spoken and unspoken sentiments, creating a bond that's fortified not just by words, but by shared experiences.

Our journey hasn't stopped at words alone. The transformative power of physical fitness and nutrition has shown us how intricately our bodies interact with our minds, painting a vivid picture of how exercise and balanced diets can stimulate not just physical health, but sexual vitality as well. Emotional intimacy, which complements these physical aspects, has emerged as crucial. Trust and vulnerability are the pillars on which deep connections are built. When partners feel safe and valued, their connection deepens, leading to a flourishing of both passion and personal satisfaction.

Moreover, we have addressed common barriers to libido, from managing stress and work-life balance to overcoming the impact of lifestyle choices. These sections offered practical solutions, reinforcing the idea that personal and shared happiness requires dedication and conscious effort. Whether undertaking challenges like stress management or opting for lifestyle adjustments, decisions made with intention can significantly enhance relational satisfaction.

The realm of sexual techniques expanded our horizons, inspiring a sense of playfulness and adventure. Experimentation in the bedroom can create an atmosphere of novelty and excitement, rekindling the flames of passion even in the most established relationships. Long-term partners have especially benefited from learning how romantic gestures and surprises can keep the spark alive, demonstrating that love is as much about commitment as it is about continual rediscovery.

Recognizing the intricacies of mental health and hormonal balance has given us a newfound appreciation for the complex interplay between our bodies and minds. Seeking help through therapy or exploring treatment options for hormonal imbalances wasn't just about addressing concerns; it was about empowering each partner to understand their unique needs and how these can affect desire and intimacy.

Our conversations with experts and real-life couples have provided valuable insights and practical advice, illustrating the power of shared experiences and the diverse approaches to intimacy enhancement. These narratives underscore the idea that while every couple's journey is unique, the road to a fulfilling intimate life is paved with shared understanding and mutual respect.

The influence of technology, stages of life, societal norms, and cultural backgrounds have been acknowledged as forces shaping our sexual desire and relationships. By acknowledging these influences, we've opened up possibilities to embrace diversity and inclusivity, understanding that love transcends boundaries and manifests differently for everyone. This awareness enriches the tapestry of our relationships, allowing us to cultivate a genuine connection that's authentically ours.

Emphasizing self-care and self-love has reminded us that nurturing one's own well-being is integral to maintaining a healthy desire. By exploring holistic approaches, such as mind-body connections, we've learned the importance of staying attuned to our needs and desires, cultivating a balance that complements our shared journey.

As we conclude our exploration, it's clear that the path to enhancing intimacy and passion is continuous and evolving. Love, in its truest form, thrives on the willingness to grow, adapt, and nurture mutual understanding. The tools and knowledge shared in this book are not finite answers but rather starting points for ongoing discovery and intimacy.

In closing, remember that the heart of intimacy lies in the journey of two souls striving to understand, respect, and cherish one another. May the insights and practices explored here serve as a guide to continually nurture your relationship, celebrating the unique bond that only you and your partner share. Here's to embracing the journey of love, in all its facets, and discovering endless possibilities together.

Appendix A:
Appendix

In this appendix, and as you embark on a journey to enhance your libido and deepen the connection with your partner, we've compiled an array of invaluable resources aimed at enriching your understanding and experience. You'll find a carefully curated selection of further readings that delve into various aspects of desire, passion, and intimate relationships. These materials include books, articles, and online content by renowned experts in the field, offering fresh perspectives and advanced insights to support this intimate voyage. Additionally, we've provided helpful contact information for professionals and support networks, empowering you to seek personalized guidance when needed. Whether you're looking to explore new dimensions of your relationship or simply deepen the ones you already cherish, this section serves as a trusted companion, guiding you with wisdom, compassion, and inspiration toward fulfilling love and intimacy.

Resources and Further Reading

In your journey toward rekindling desire and fostering an enriching intimate relationship, a wealth of resources can guide you. As you strive for an enhanced connection with your partner, exploring reputable books, articles, and online platforms can be immensely beneficial. These resources collectively offer practical guidance, expert insights, and the personal experiences of individuals who've navigated similar paths.

One invaluable resource is *"Come as You Are: The Surprising New Science That Will Transform Your Sex Life"* by Emily Nagoski. This book uncovers the science of desire through real-life stories and practical advice, encouraging a deeper understanding of personal sexuality. It's a compelling read for anyone looking to enhance their intimacy and connect emotionally with their partner.

Another significant work is *"The Passionate Marriage: Keeping Love and Intimacy Alive in Committed Relationships"* by David Schnarch. The book delves into building emotional connections and maintaining passion in long-term relationships. It discusses the psychological underpinnings of desire and provides strategies to overcome emotional barriers.

For those interested in the interplay of physical fitness and libido, *"Spark: The Revolutionary New Science of Exercise and the Brain"* by John Ratey explores how physical activity can enhance cognitive functions and libido. It's an enlightening resource for understanding how exercise can positively affect your relationship.

If you're keen on exploring self-care in enhancing intimacy, consider *"Radical Acceptance: Embracing Your Life With the Heart of a Buddha"* by Tara Brach. This book emphasizes the importance of accepting oneself and others, promoting personal well-being as a critical component of intimate relationships.

The field of nutritional science offers research papers on how diet influences libido and energy levels. Search for journals such as the *Journal of Sexual Medicine* or the *American Journal of Clinical Nutrition* to access scholarly articles about the impact of nutrition on sexual health.

There are also numerous online platforms and forums that discuss intimacy and desire. Websites like *Lovehoney* or *Good in Bed* provide a community-based approach, where individuals can share personal experiences, tips, and advice on maintaining an exciting intimate life. These communities can be supportive environments to learn from others' experiences.

Further exploration into mental health services, such as therapy and counseling, can be beneficial. Organizations like the *American Psychological Association* and *Mental Health America* provide directories and resources for finding a therapist specializing in relationship and sexual health.

Podcasts focusing on relationships, intimacy, and sexual health can be a modern and accessible way to gain insights. Programs like *"Where Should We Begin?"* with Esther Perel offer an engaging approach to learning about relationship dynamics from the perspective of a renowned therapist.

Consider documentaries that explore themes of love, intimacy, and human connection. Films such as *"The Nature of Love"* or *"Love Me"* provide a visual and narrative exploration of romantic relationships and the complexities inherent in maintaining passion over time.

As societal perspectives continue to evolve, books addressing cultural impacts on intimacy, like *"The Sexual Healing Journey: A Guide for Survivors of Sexual Abuse"* by Wendy Maltz, can offer valuable insights for those dealing with past trauma. Understanding cultural and personal history is key to liberating current desires and intimacy.

Education is ongoing, and attending workshops or seminars can enrich your understanding of desire and intimacy. Look for events curated by organizations such as *The Gottman Institute* or *Sexual*

Health Alliance, where experts provide evidence-based strategies for improving relationship satisfaction.

Lastly, holistic approaches can resonate with those interested in mind-body-spirit connections. Books like *"The Body Keeps the Score: Brain, Mind, and Body in the Healing of Trauma"* by Bessel van der Kolk provide comprehensive exploration on how psychological health intertwines with physical experiences, helping couples understand the full spectrum of intimacy.

In summary, numerous resources, from scholarly journals to best-selling books, podcasts, and online communities, can support your journey. They offer diverse perspectives to enrich your understanding of intimacy and desire, aiding you in cultivating a fulfilling love life. Always keep an open mind and explore various materials and platforms to discover what resonates with you and your partner.

Helpful Contact Information

In the journey of enhancing your libido and deepening intimacy, knowing where to turn for support can be invaluable. This section provides a comprehensive list of contacts and resources that can serve as a guiding light as you navigate through various aspects of your relationship. The professional guidance, support groups, and educational materials listed here are intended to offer assistance whenever you need a helping hand, a listening ear, or an expert opinion.

Seeking professional advice is often the first step many couples take when addressing intimacy issues. The American Association of Sexuality Educators, Counselors, and Therapists (**AASECT**) offers a database of certified professionals specializing in sexual health and intimacy. Whether you're looking for a therapist for one-on-one sessions or a counselor to guide you and your partner through challenges, AASECT professionals provide quality care that respects your unique needs.

The *Society for Sex Therapy and Research* (**SSTAR**) is another commendable organization you can turn to for locating experienced and well-trained sex therapists. SSTAR's mission is to advance the understanding of human sexuality, and they provide a platform for finding professionals committed to ethical and effective therapy. This can be particularly helpful if you're seeking therapy from those with a strong academic and research-backed foundation.

An often overlooked but crucial aspect of maintaining intimacy and libido is addressing underlying health issues. For this, consider reaching out to the **National Institute of Health**'s department specializing in sexual health. Their educational resources focus on the biological and psychological intricacies of libido, offering you a wealth of information directly from leaders in medical research.

For couples interested in natural and holistic approaches, the *American Herbalists Guild* can be a valuable resource. They have an extensive directory of certified herbalists who specialize in using plant-based remedies to enhance libido and improve overall health. Engaging with a registered herbalist can help you incorporate safe and effective supplements into your routine.

Community support plays a significant role in navigating the sometimes rocky path of intimacy enhancement. Consider joining online forums or local support groups, such as those found on the *Reddit Communities* tailored to relationship advice or intimacy discussions. Engaging with a community allows you to share experiences and receive encouragement and insights from others facing similar challenges. These platforms foster a sense of belonging, reminding you that you are not alone in this journey.

In this digital age, technology offers innovative solutions for intimacy. Apps like **Lasting** focus on improving relationships through guided communication exercises. While not a substitute for therapy, they offer practical tools for strengthening your bond and understanding between partners. Try to explore digital tools that align with your values and goals, helping you maintain a balance in your intimate life.

If you're struggling with mental health issues affecting your libido, reaching out to the **National Alliance on Mental Illness** (**NAMI**) can provide essential support. They offer free classes and support groups for those dealing with mental health crises or conditions. Understanding and addressing mental health is crucial for a healthy intimate relationship, as a balanced mind directly influences desire and connection.

For those who'd rather delve into academic and experiential learning, attending workshops or retreats can be an enlightening experience. Organizations such as **Esalen Institute** offer immersive workshops on intimacy, communication, and partnership. These retreats provide a safe space for personal and relational growth, encouraging deeper connections in serene, transformative environments.

Lastly, keeping abreast of new research and findings in sexuality and intimacy can empower you to take informed steps in your journey. Subscribing to industry journals, like the *Journal of Sex & Marital Therapy*, ensures you have access to contemporary discussions, studies, and expert opinions on sexual health.

Combining these resources, you're strategically equipped to tackle any barriers in enhancing your libido and intimate connection. Whether seeking professional guidance or community support, these contacts provide a steady support network. Remember, reaching out for help is a strength, and pursuing a fulfilling love life is a profound and noble endeavor.

www.ingramcontent.com/pod-product-compliance
Lightning Source LLC
Chambersburg PA
CBHW030302290526
45785CB00001B/179